"The great irony is that as women arguably e[...] of contribution, they are also plagued by th[e] malaise of menopause.

I've known Tracy my whole adult life, and she's always been that girl. That girl who always said yes and found a way through. That girl with an insatiable curiosity. That girl seeking a path less trodden. That girl with a massive work ethic. That girl with her shit together. Until she didn't.

And this is what makes this book all the more powerful. My Menopause Memoir is a stumble through Tracy's B-roll as her shit came unstuck. Her deeply personal journey through menopause, as, along with her sisterhood, Tracy plots, what can be, a relentless march through the 35 known symptoms of peri, meno, and post-menopause – from hot flashes to considering HRT – the war on our physical, mental, and emotional equilibrium – in essence, losing who we are.

But more importantly – Tracy shares the next steps in the path back. Part lifestyle, part intervention - Tracy fosters a healthy respect for medical research, lifestyle hacks, and pragmatic self-experiment.

My Menopause Memoir is an invitation for ladies of a particular age and phase, and all those around them, to see themselves in the pages, to start to piece together their own summer cocktail of symptoms and to explore remedies to balance themselves again.

Alongside the Sexy Ageing Podcast, this body of work forms the basis of an evolving conversation to demystify what past generations had to endure and to normalize how future generations will respond.

Take a leaf from Tracy's book. Know that you are not alone. Listen. Talk. Share. Try stuff."

Emma Barry
Global Fitness Authority | Co-founder – Good Soul Hunting |
Senior Advisor – FitTech Company
Friend | Colleague | Fellow Physeder
Ibiza Forever

"Tracy's memoir captures true emotion associated with a normal life transition for someone, who despite being self aware, felt it came as a complete surprise. Tracy has spent a lifetime striving to be natural and in tune with her mind and body but despite having these skills she needed to *delve into the science to understand these new changes. Now, supported by her new knowledge of the latest evidence in mid-life medicine and still notexperiencing the quality of life she knew she could achieve, she explains how hormone replacement therapy is safe, effective, body-identical and still aligns with her values. And fundamentally it provided the symptom improvement she needed to live her life as she wishes. Her quest to explore the physiological changes associated with menopause is supported by poignant stories from other women which will resonate with the readers experience."*

Samantha K Newman
MBChB BSc (hons)
Founder of femaleGP, NZ
Director of Newman Medical Services

"My Menopause Memoir takes the topic of menopause that often has shame and embarrassment associated with it, and turns it into a discussion that empowers women and their bodies. Tracy adds much needed humor to the subject to make us all feel 'normal' and her personal stories shine through to entertain and educate all and let us know we are aren't alone. It's a must read not only for all women, but also their partners and families to truly understand this important life stage, and the impact it can have on our daily lives."

Natalie Dau
Creator of Rockstar Fit and Host of Zero to Hero TV

MY MENOPAUSE MEMOIR

FROM THE FOUNDER OF SEXY AGEING PODCAST

BY TRACY MINNOCH-NUKU

COPYRIGHT

Copyright © 2022 by Tracy Minnoch-Nuku, Tauranga, New Zealand

All rights reserved. No part of this publication may be reproduced in any form, or by any means, electronic or mechanical, including photocopying, recording, or any information browsing, storage, or retrieval system, without permission in writing from the author.

Although this publication is designed to provide accurate information in regard to the subject matter covered, the author assumes no responsibility for the changing landscape of the science and health studies that provide future up-to-date information and data on this subject matter. This publication is meant as a source of valuable information for the reader, however it is not meant as a replacement for direct expert assistance. If such level of assistance is required, the services of a competent professional should be sought.

www.sexyageing.com
First Edition, 2022
First Printing, 2022

Author Photograph: Sarah Grasett

DEDICATION

I dedicate this book to my children, Jazz and Sol, so they might have the menopause conversation as a normal and daily part of their lives.

CONTENTS

Prologue 1
Sleep challenges 9
Fatigue 19
Hot flashes 23
Night Sweats 25
Sore feet and leg cramps 31
Joint pain 35
Tight muscles 39
Irregular periods 41
Brain fog 45
Memory loss 51
Stress 57
Mood swings and anxiety 61
Lacking motivation 67
Bloating and digestive issues 69
Inflammation 73
Losing libido 79
Incontinence 83
Breast pain 87
Acne 89
Dry, itchy skin 93
Dry eyes 95
Hair loss (and gain) 99
Brittle nails 103
Body odour 107
Heart palpitations 111
Dizziness 115
Electric shocks 119
Allergies 121
Co-ordination 123
Weight gain 125
Chills 129
Vaginal dryness 131
Headaches 135
Burning mouth syndrome 137

Gum problems and dental issues 139
Epilogue 143
Acknowledgements 145
About the author 147
Recommended resources 149

PROLOGUE

Eight months ago, I tentatively launched a podcast called "Sexy Ageing" with the prospect of initiating discussions with women and men and understand what the ageing process means to them. The conversations cover everything from hormonal health to starting a new business and the midlife growth mindset. The podcast aims to educate and inspire, and I'm so grateful for the guests who have shared their experiences and for the listeners who have responded positively. Every time I go for a run or a walk with my husband Dave, we inevitably talk about what's happening with my Sexy Ageing podcast, the feedback I have had from a listener or a conversation I've had with my sister or a friend about their experience with THE MENOPAUSE. A common theme is how they are struggling to communicate their symptoms and experience to their health provider. Dave encouraged me to write it down because it's a lot to take in and "how are other women coping with all of this if we are constantly exploring another new symptom?"

So here I am, awake at 4am and committed to getting my thoughts down on paper. All I think about, and sometimes dream about, is perimenopause and menopause. How to share what I'm experiencing with other women? And men! It's a LOT. It's confusing, sometimes debilitating, isolating and yet, here we are. An army of women shouting that we need to do better in supporting our midlife women through this journey to source accurate, simple and practical information on how to manage the changes that are happening to our bodies, that messes with our minds and our emotions and leaves us feeling strung out, wrung out and alone.

I'm one of those women who will lay it all out there, but not before I've researched the situation because I don't like to provide inaccurate information. My search for answers to what midlife and beyond could look like started from a place of vanity, to be honest. When I turned 45,

I started to visualise what my life would be like when I was in my 50's. I knew that I wanted to bust any myths about what life "should" be for a midlife woman, and create something different for myself.

For my 45th birthday, my friend Kym gifted me "The Longevity Book" by Cameron Diaz. It sat on my book shelf for a few months before I picked it up and began to wade into the science of ageing. I read case studies of how the body ages and how some people have lived to be 100 or more. I was inspired. I don't remember the book having much information on hormonal changes for women, but the idea that I could have a long healthy life by making some positive changes to my lifestyle left a lasting impression.

I wanted to know more and experience a vibrant life every day. I went down the rabbit hole, like many of us do when we start to explore a topic that is new to us and one that we know will help us reap the personal benefits. More books, podcasts, YouTube, investigating those that reside in the Blue Zone countries and how they live longer than anyone else. Then shit hit the fan. Unusual and unexpected events began to mess with my body and mind. Sleeplessness, night sweats, anxiety, fatigue, forgetfulness, a loss in confidence, inexplicable rage and more. I couldn't understand what was happening to me. It took 18 months of personal research to finally see the word that might explain my experience - menopause.

For the benefit of anyone who has not yet bumped up against the world of menopause, let me break it down for you because you do not need Latin for this one. *Meno* is your menstrual cycle. *Pause* is, of course, to stop. But menopause isn't just one phase that happens for all women. It's broken down into a series of events and symptoms and can begin, for some, as early as their 30's.

Premenopause: you aren't experiencing any changes to your menstrual cycle and you haven't noticed any strange or unexpected symptoms.

Perimenopause: this is the time the effects of your fluctuating hormones become more noticeable. Perhaps you're experiencing heavier or irregular periods, sleep disruptions, hot flashes, night sweats or weight gain. These are the most common reported symptoms from women. This stage can last anywhere from 4 to 10 years and for some women, even longer. That is potentially a whole decade of your life in which you have to deal with some gnarly shit.

Menopause: This is the general word used for all the things that have happened to bring you to this point but in actual fact, menopause is just ONE day - the day you have not had a menstrual period for 12 months.

Postmenopause: Everything that follows once your period stops falls into this category. This means no more PMS or periods - yahoo! No more birth control and most perimenopausal symptoms will subside, but you will need to become vigilant to your heart, brain and bone health.

Surgical Menopause: it is common for menopause symptoms to kick start if you have had your ovaries surgically removed[1]. And the symptoms of menopause are often quicker and more pronounced.

If you're feeling somewhat overwhelmed, and possibly disappointed that you haven't been told any of this prior to experiencing symptoms, then you are in the the majority of women globally. According to the medical sources, 1.2 billion women will be in menopause by 2030.[2] And if you are 30+ and an enlightened friend has highly recommended you read this, then consider it an investment in your future health. Irrespective of where you are at today, view this memoir as a tool kit for your evolving hormonal journey.

Bolstered by the conversations I had with friends, family and through my podcast, I was motivated to get ahead of what happens to a women during menopause. I studied and completed courses on Healthy Ageing for Midlife Women with a specific focus on health and fitness training. I have applied as much of the science to myself as possible with a view to support my menopause transition. So many of the changes I have made have been positive and I felt better over time. Some of the changes still require my attention. This book has been written so you can learn about this life transition through my personal experiences and the experience of some amazing women who have generously shared their stories. Guest testimonies shine a light on how every women's menopause transition is different.

---

1   Such as surgery for endometriosis, cancer treatments and chemotherapy, genetic and autoimmune diseases

2   https://pubmed.ncbi.nlm.nih.gov/8735350/

According to reputable women's health resources, such as Newson Health Menopause and Wellbeing Clinic in the UK[3] and the North American Menopause Society[4], at the time of writing, there are 35 recognised menopause symptoms. I share my 29 out of 35 symptoms. Each chapter will be supported by scientific, yet easy to understand facts, and then an action list - your "to do" list of ways you can support, and in some cases alleviate the symptoms to take control of the out-of-control, making daily living that little bit easier.

---

[3] https://www.newsonhealth.co.uk
[4] https://www.menopause.org

DISCLAIMER

I am a qualified, lifelong fitness professional but I am not a medical expert and so the recommendations I have made in the book are through research, recommendations from women's health experts and through my personal experience. I have always believed that you can influence your own personal health through the foundations of movement, adequate nutrition and lifestyle factors - sleep, not smoking, a stress free existence, community and a sense of purpose. By actively seeking to make incremental improvements in any of these key areas and stay the course, medical conditions aside, you can continue to make positive changes that have a lasting impact over time.

I want to help women in the future figure out how they should be exercising for maximum fitness and wellness gains. I have made good progress on many of the symptoms that affected me daily - my sleep improved, my gut health repaired and I had a general sense of wellbeing that lasted most days. And yet, I still had niggling symptoms that annoyed me and despite all the natural methods, I wanted to explore MHT (Menopause Hormone Therapy), also known as HRT (Hormonal Replacement Therapy). I wanted to see if this would make a difference. And it did. For those symptoms, I have included where HRT helped me. So I will say, that HRT might not be the choice for everyone and I would always recommend prioritising the necessary lifestyle changes alongside HRT for best results.

When I began to think about one symptom to share my menopause experience I realised how challenging that was going to be. I had lots of symptoms. I'm not even sure which arrived on the scene first or even when they did, it just felt like once I'd come to grips with one thing, something else presented itself and sent me into another downward spiral. The lack of sleep, the mood swings, the sometimes uncontrollable rage where I really felt I could have ripped someones head off, the weight gain, (middle age spread really is a thing!) and then having to admit that no matter what I did I couldn't control any of this.

I don't even remember when it started. One minute I was sleeping soundly, getting a solid 7-8 hours sleep a night. The next I was waking up 4,5,6 times every night, sometimes sweating like I'd just taught an extended spin class, and just unbelievably hot like someone had snuck in and turned my electric blanket on. I would kick off the covers and strip off my clothes. I started leaving a cold, wet flannel on my bedside table and after draping it across me, I would wake up what seemed like only five minutes later, absolutely freezing. The lack of sleep led to the crazy mood swings, or maybe the mood swings led to the lack of sleep. WHO KNOWS?

I vividly remember locking myself in my wardrobe one day, not knowing whether to cry my heart out or pick up the keys and drive, just to get away from anyone and everyone. No one really understood what was going on in my head and no matter how hard I tried to tell them, the looks on their faces said it all. Any little thing would set me off, especially with the kids. I am a bit of neat freak and I feel terrible now when I think back to the way I reacted to the smallest thing. Hopefully one day they will understand I really, truly couldn't control myself. I tried to train harder, lift more, ride faster, walk further, do more push ups, do more sit ups - anything that would tell me I was still in control. Well, that didn't work.

I developed vertigo, varying degrees of it, maybe brought about by lack of sleep, maybe just another menopause gift when you google it, another possible symptom. I stopped drinking coffee, the vertigo stopped and I haven't touched a drop in over 4 years, too scared now to even have one.

It was tough. I felt like I was dealing with this alone. I lost my Mum in 2011. Mum was advised to have a hysterectomy quite early in her life. The male specialist said, "Well if you're not planning on having more children, does it really make a difference?".Mum always regretted that decision. She also had a terrible time with the HRT drugs that she was prescribed, so all those things were on my mind.I just wanted to talk with her and it brought back my loss even more and the emotional roller coaster I was on just got more and more out of control. Amongst all of this, the problems I had been having with my voice escalated and I thought well, maybe it is better if I don't voice my problems and just learn to deal with it by myself. That was tough. I had always loved going out and being with people. I love a good party, but what was the use when no one could hear me. I know now my voice probably wasn't related to my menopause but at the time it was a good excuse.

Just as I can't quite tell you when it all started, I really can't quite remember when I started to regain control either.I started journaling. I changed quite a few things in my diet. I got back into reading and taking time to actually do nothing and not feel guilty about that. I started to sleep better, which for me made a huge difference. Strange though, the last few months, I have started getting hot flushes again, nothing like before but enough to wake me in the night. I know listening to the Sexy Ageing podcasts has helped me realise we are all the same, we all have these thoughts, we are all dealing with this 'shit that is menopause' and somehow that makes it easier to deal with.

Stella MacGregor,
New Zealand

SLEEP CHALLENGES

Do you know that amazing feeling when you get into bed, fall right asleep, stay asleep all night, and wake up feeling refreshed? Yeah, me neither… I wake up. It's 2amish. I lie in bed tossing around and think I will probably fall asleep again in a few minutes. 20 mins….45 mins….60 mins…. WTF! Get up. Go downstairs, make a herbal tea and open up my laptop. I am literally cringing as I write this because if I only knew NOT to open my laptop, if only I could have had that knowledge and self control.

The herbal tea is nice. The house is quiet. I can't even remember what I was doing on the laptop. Probably nothing productive. 4am. Feeling a bit sleepy. Go back to bed. The air-conditioning is powering on and I fall asleep. 6am. Alarm goes off. Feel like I've been hit by a truck. Get up and get through the day. It was just ONE bad sleep, right?

Next night. Same situation. I am now catatonic. I was so tired when I went to bed. I thought I would sleep like the dead but now I am awake again at 2am. What is this witchery? Am I subconsciously preparing for an all night dance party? I get up sooner and grab a book this time. If I am going to be awake, me and my tea, then I will fill my mind with a story and fatigue my eyes.

This went off and on for 18 months, before I even considered to investigate a reason for sleeplessness. Even while I was on holiday, away from the stress and to-do lists, I was waking at the same time. I decided to tap into Dr Google. This was the first time I came across the word "perimenopause". I have a few older female friends and no one ever mentioned this or any other symptoms they were experiencing. My doctor had never spoken of it when we decided that the Mirena IUS at 45 years old would be a good way to continue with contraception. In my sleep deprived state that had started to cause even more issues, I felt let down and confused as to why no one had even mentioned that I should know what perimenopause was.

40-60% of women in the menopause transition report sleep disturbances.[5] Quality sleep can help to ward off other symptoms but then here we are, the ultimate Catch-22 needing sleep but not being able to!

---

[5] Source: Krause AJ, Simon EB, Mander BA, Greer SM, Saletin JM, Goldstein-Piekarski AN, Walker MP. The sleep-deprived human brain. Nat Rev Neurosci. 2017 Jul;18(7):404-418.

"My absolute worst menopause symptom has been insomnia and it was the first symptom that presented during perimenopause and continues to be a daily battle. I had chronic fatigue for 15 years and I used to joke that I could sleep on a washing line but when "menosomnia" hit, I just couldn't sleep at all. Its effect on me meant that for a year, I couldn't work. I had to try to sleep at various times of the day because I might not be able to sleep until 6am. It meant I didn't have the ability to book anything into my diary. I felt like I was a zombie, the walking dead most of the day because I was absolutely exhausted.

I had virtually no help from any doctors - actually that's unfair - they gave me everything they could. I was given amitriptyline (an anti-depressant), CBT (Cognitive Behavioural Therapy), told to learn a new language in the time I was awake but I was just exhausted all the time. My brain wouldn't function, my fitness went out the window. It was absolutely horrendous. A GP had told me to give up working which wasn't going to happen as a single, self-employed mother who spent fourteen years getting to the peak of my career. The amitriptyline stopped working. I ended up trying to access valium wherever I could, just to be able to have a night or two of sleep.

What I've learnt is I've had to be incredibly strict with my diet - if I have alcohol, my sleep goes out the window. If I am nervous, anxious or scared, my sleep is disrupted. I have worked with sleep psychiatrists, taken up meditation, counselling, exercise - everything is planned to help me get to a place of having a good nights' sleep. My partner and I mostly have to sleep in separate rooms. I HAVE to be in bed by 10pm with the lights out and it usually takes me about an hour to fall asleep.

Through all of this, I have learnt a lot about myself. I have learnt that I am resilient, and to surrender - I have this communication with my body where I tell it what the next day is going to involve and I trust it to get the sleep it needs to be able to function. And some days when I get 5-6 hours sleep, I can kick ass and not be jacked up on coffee. It also got better when I found the right hormones for me - I'm using a natural sublingual progesterone and that really helps.

Through all this, I came to the realisation that I had never presented as an anxious person. Anxiety is hidden in me. It's very deep and I have learnt how to work with that. I have learnt so much about myself and that REST is the most important thing. I have to schedule time everyday for exercise and rest time between meetings. I allow myself, even if it's just for 20 minutes to lie in a dark room, just in case I hadn't slept well the night before. I have had to learn to prioritise self care and that has been a blessing. The message that I have learnt from the menopause transition is to prioritise ourselves to be able to function for those that need us."

Claire Snowdon-Darling,
UK (Hormones and Emotions Expert)

"Sleep - lack of, late onset, shit sleep. This has been one of the most annoying symptoms that I am experiencing in my early stage of peri-menopause. I have an autoimmune disease and anyone who has the same would completely appreciate how important sleep is in managing symptoms and controlling the disease. While I have been journalling my sleep for a while and applying structured sleep hygiene, I still wasn't getting the benefits from doing that.

I've spoken with my doctor who has started me on melatonin supplementation, which is fantastic. I'm not a candidate (yet) for HRT because of the complexity of my medical condition. Melatonin is not funded in New Zealand which feels like another barrier to women, or anyone who needs to have good sleep.

Through the Sexy Ageing podcast episodes and the information shared by so many of the guests who have all experienced this symptom, it's obviously not such a phenomena and people are talking about it. This has empowered me to feel the confidence to explore HOW to address the symptoms, get on top of them and not accept them as the way things will be from here on."

Tia Minnoch,
New Zealand (Clinical Nurse Specialist)

The changes happening to our bodies, specifically the hormonal changes, are responsible for so many of the symptoms that show up as we transition through menopause. The disruption of sleep has a heightened and flow on affect to many of the symptoms I was personally experiencing. When I speak to others about some of the challenges they are experiencing with their menopause transition, lack of sleep is often a conversation starter.

As we age, magical melatonin, the hormone responsible for our sleep-wake cycle, begins to taper off, resulting in sleep disruption. Put that together with dropping oestrogen and progesterone and you have a potent mix for that all night dance party.

Melatonin is responsible for more than our circadian rhythms - blood pressure, body temperature and the release of other hormones can also be affected. Understanding this about my body, I began sleep tracking, which requires using a sleep tracker or wearing a smart watch to bed. The daily data and trends helped me to understand the importance of the sleep cycle and the optimum amount of sleep needed for my gender and stage of life. I learnt what quality sleep meant and which activities will cause a bad nights sleep.

When I began to use the sleep tracking app and added the specifics for my gender, age and activity levels, I could see the sleep cycle targets I should be aiming for and the patterns in my own sleep, or lack of. The sleep tracker begins to record data once you lie down in bed. The descriptions and targets for a sleep cycle are provided with my personal metrics.

While sleeping, we experience a series of "sleep cycles" that comprise of REM - rapid eye movement - and non-REM sleep.

REM sleep is associated with dreaming and usually has the most impact at the back end your sleep. REM sleep is for mental restoration, converting short term memories into long term ones. This would be likened to backing up your memory on your computer or smartphone. The goal for REM sleep is 15-25% of total time sleeping.

For non-REM Sleep ,there are 3 stages and some baseline goals for a 50 year old woman .For example ,if you aim to consistently reach 7 hours of sleep per night.

- Stage - 1 between awake and asleep .The recommended target is 12-24%of total sleep time ,or between 1.5 - 1 hours.

- Stage - 2 light sleep where your body temperature and heart rate lowers and breathing regulates .The target is for 40-60% of total time asleep ,between 4 - 3 hours.
- Stage - 3 Deep Sleep gives physical and mental restoration .Aim for 8-16% of total time asleep ,between 1.5 - 1 hours sleep.

The most common time to wake for perimenopausal women is between 2.00 - 4.00am when REM sleep is starting to lengthen. Being awake during 1-2 sleep cycles affects the brain's ability to "back up". Over time, the negative impact to your life include forgetfulness, brain fog, fatigue and feeling impatient, or just fucked off, to put it bluntly.

Consistently waking up through the night will wreck havoc on your hormones. That 2.00am - 4.00am window is where you need to be sleeping for hormone regulation and avoid the fall out from further perimenopause affects. You want to be asleep but your changing hormone production is keeping you awake.

Here is a list of the hormones and the changes:

Decreasing Melatonin - Melatonin regulates our sleep-wake cycle. Melatonin naturally decreases with age.

Increasing Cortisol - This hormone increases with age and stress.

Decreasing Seratonin - Our "happy hormone" decreases as we age, which is linked to feelings of heightened anxiety and/or depression.

Decreasing Oestrogen - Having less oestrogen makes it harder to fall asleep and stay asleep, and has a direct impact on serotonin levels. Less oestrogen means less serotonin. Falling oestrogen levels affect body temperature regulation as well. Cue hot flashes and night sweats.

Decreasing Progesterone - Progesterone helps us to relax. Decreasing levels of progesterone produce less of a sedative affect.

Insulin and Cortisol - Higher levels of insulin and cortisol in the body will slow down overnight fat burning and make it harder for melatonin to help you rest and sleep. Hence the correlation between poor sleep and increasing fat, particularly to the belly.

If after reading and digesting all these facts on hormones and how they effect your sleep, you may be thinking that there is no hope - but hang in there! If we focus on this symptom FIRST, we can successfully support some of the other symptoms that align themselves with perimenopause.

TIPS FOR SUPPORTING SLEEP DISRUPTION

If you are reading this chapter and feeling the frustration at not being able to sleep through the night, I feel you. I got you. That sensation of half-functioning throughout the day and all the other fallouts from a sleepless night are debilitating. Here are a list of things you could try and gradually make daily conscious changes for the betterment of your life in this next stage. I recommend that you start with one or two of the suggestions below that feel easy to implement, and then gradually add on more, as some of these tips will challenge aspects of your current lifestyle.

- Prioritise your natural rhythm. Working longer hours, staying up later and watching TV well into the night are messing with our body's circadian rhythm. Melatonin production relies on our body to wake up and go to sleep at the optimal times. Waking up with the sun (6-7am) and getting outside into the natural light, when possible, optimises our master internal clock.
- At night, reduce screen time or "blue light". This is another inhibitor of melatonin production. Using blue-light blocking glasses, the night setting on your devices and shutting down devices 60-90 minutes before going to bed can improve the quality of your sleep.
- The goal is to get 7-9 hours of quality sleep based on the stages and optimal recommendations for your age and gender. Using a sleep tracker will help you understand what is happening on a nightly basis. It will only take two weeks of data before you notice the correlations in quality, quantity and how you feel throughout the day.
- Leading up to bedtime, switch off all devices or move away from the laptop/TV/iPad. This really does mean that you won't be watching Netflix or any device driven entertainment from bed. I have to be so disciplined with this during the work week as my

sleep quality was obviously impacted with device use versus reading a book before lights out. I do enjoy the weekends for Netflix catch ups though.
- Your bedtime ritual - and I do mean ritual. A conscious play-by-play checklist that you implement to relax your body and mind. It can be really challenging to follow through on the list when you have work and home to-do lists that flow into your evenings. The work deadline that now requires your attention after everyone else has gone to bed, the laundry that needs folding, the bills that need to be paid. I know it! One thing I have mastered the art of through the years is delegation. Recruit the family members to decrease your to-do list and explain nicely that they will enjoy a "loving, kind and all about them mum" versus "bitch, psychotic killer mum" when they can help you tackle the to-do list so you can get to bed at a reasonable hour. If your family have been on the receiving end of psycho-mum too many times, then they don't need an explanation as to why they are now folding the laundry on Tuesdays and Thursdays.
- Caffeine - 2 cups maximum per day, both before 12pm.
- Exercise - if you are planning a hard workout, get it done before midday. More gentle movement such as walks and slow flow yoga are better later in the day. Cortisol levels are at their highest after waking up and cortisol also spikes through high intensity exercise. This doesn't help if you want to sleep, so allow your cortisol levels to decrease throughout the day and set yourself up for a better chance of quality sleep.
- No naps - try not to nap during the day. We are trying to regulate our circadian rhythms and a nap, unless you've had no sleep the night before or are ill, will mess with that.
- Alcohol really screws with sleep quality. The best nights to focus on getting quality sleep is Sunday - Friday so try to abstain until the weekend and then stop drinking before 7.00pm. Unless it's a celebration - then go for it! I'm not a kill-joy! Those special moments in life that require celebration are important. If you have been using a sleep tracker, you will see a direct correlation between sleep quality and alcohol consumption.
- Nutrition Tips: avoid spicy and acidic foods at night. Include high quality carbohydrates such as sweet potato, brown rice, lentils and

quinoa. I have strong science based views on nutrition, and depriving yourself of healthy, complex carbohydrates is not optimal, at any stage of life.
- Set yourself a timer to remind you it's time to wind down and shut down your devices 60-90 minutes before you plan to go to bed.
- Put away everything - a quick tidy up and prepping your bedroom for sleep gets you in the mood.
- Make a list of priorities for the next day. Write it down.
- And while you are writing, list 3-5 things you are grateful for! You know all the science about that so no preaching here.
- Set up your bedroom candle or diffuser, or both. Research tells us that the "inhalation of lavender essential oil is a safe, low-cost practice that should be considered as a complementary option to conventional treatments, whether medical, psychological or other integrative and complementary practices" [6]
- Try a simple and relaxing 10-15 minute yoga practice or stretches followed by 5-10 minutes of meditation. This is physically and mentally preparing your wind down.
- Taking a warm and relaxing bath or shower. I found that when I lived in the tropics, it was better for my body to have a tepid shower and lower my body temperature but now that I'm back in New Zealand with four seasons, that hot shower sure feels good in the cold of winter.
- If possible, lower the temperature of your bedroom to around 18C or 65F. If you aren't able to manipulate your room temperature, ensure that you have cool cotton sheets and/or a bamboo blanket.
- Use blackout curtains to enhance that circadian rhythm, blocking out any street light.
- Read - whether it's 15 minutes or up until light's out.
- Night Time Herbal Teas: any combination of chamomile, passionflower, lemon balm, lavender, oatflower, lime flower, liquorice root and valerian root are a great addition to your bedtime routine

---

6   0498 Effect of Lavender Essential Oil on Sleep in Postmenopausal Women with Insomnia: Double-Blind Randomized Controlled Trial

L R Lucena, J G Santos-Junior, S Tufik, H Hachul

Sleep, Volume 43, Issue Supplement_1, April 2020, Pages A190–A191, https://doi.org/10.1093/sleep/zsaa056.495

Published: 27 May 2020

I know this seems like a lot to get you ready for bed and quality sleep. The key is to choose some practices and see how those work for you. Start with the tips that feel the most natural to you and repeat those for 5-7 days. Then add on one more if you feel you can improve further.

I can't say with 100% certainty whether HRT improved my sleep or not, as by the time I had started using it, I had an excellent bedtime routine which provided me with good quality sleep. My personal opinion leans towards doing what you can from the list above as these are healthy and lifelong recommendations that will make great improvements to your symptoms overall. If HRT is not an option, then maximising these recommendations should be a priority.

RECOMMENDED SLEEP SUPPORT SUPPLEMENTS

- Magnesium glycinate, 400-600mg 60 minutes before bedtime. Look for the "glycinate" version as it is able to cross the blood-brain barrier, affects the bowels less and is better for sleep, mood and migraines.
- Melatonin: In New Zealand, it is possible to get a prescription for 2mg. This is a regulated supplement. Take 60 minutes before bedtime.
- Vitamin B6/B12: has been shown to boost serotonin levels[7]. Vitamin B6 can be prescribed by your GP and the recommended dosage is 25-50mg/day while being mindful of the levels of B6 in other supplements taken.

---

7   The Effects of Magnesium – Melatonin - Vit B Complex Supplementation in Treatment of Insomnia
Open Access Maced J Med Sci. 2019 Sep 30; 7(18): 3101–3105.
Published online 2019 Aug 30. doi:10.3889/oamjms.2019.771
https://www.ncbi.nlm.nih.gov/pmc/articles/PMC6910806/

FATIGUE

It makes a lot of sense that if you aren't sleeping you will experience fatigue. Even when I did manage to catch up on some sleep, I constantly felt like I was never able to fully function. I could say that it was the "natural" ageing process and maybe that is acceptable when it comes to physical ageing to a degree, but when the fatigue began to effect my motivation for doing things, going out, meeting friends, checking off the "to do" list, I was left with a despairing sense that life was all downhill from here. Without fully understanding what was going on, I started to double down on my detail to sleep tracking and ensuring that if I was missing hours one night, I would go to bed earlier the next night to make up for it.

I focused on winding down the amount and intensity of physical exercise and became very attentive to when and how I would train my body. I had experienced adrenal fatigue in my early 40's so I knew the negative impact of too much cortisol and adrenaline flowing around my system. I was terrified that over training of any kind would set me back on that path. The irony was that during the time of my worst peri-menopausal symptoms of sleep loss and fatigue, I was working on new fitness programs across our business AND a fitness app. I was constantly churning out content, training, rehearsing, teaching. My fitness friends were always encouraging me to join this class, enter this run, do another workout and it left me slammed.

I began to gravitate more towards my yoga practice, as each and every time I practiced or taught a class, I could feel an immense relief in my body - like every cell and fibre was thanking me.

One of the worst impacts of fatigue is that end of day feeling where all you can think about is getting dinner over and done with and crawling into bed. This becomes a cycle and starts to impact on your motivation to go out, meet friends, try new activities, pick up a new hobby, learn something new, or even just call people for a chat. And you can see why midlife women start to hibernate or draw into themselves. Life just gets too hard.

At this point, after years of research and finally talking to one of the leading doctors in menopause care, Dr Rebecca Lewis from Newson Health UK, I decided to bite the bullet and try HRT (hormonal replacement therapy).

After 3 days with my first oestrogen patch, I can hand-on-heart say that fatigue was the first symptom that improved. I felt focused, motivated and could fully function right to the end of the day. It just goes to show that women who are no longer trapped in the sleep loss cycle and feel like they have their mojo back, can resume exercise or yoga or meditation, make better food choices and reconnect with friends.

Fatigue in your 40's is not solely attributed to perimenopause and/or menopause symptoms. It could also be low thyroid function, low B12 and folic acid, nutritional deficiencies, low iron and anaemia, so it's ideal to have a blood test to rule out any of these.

Just a Vitamin B12 deficiency alone can bring on fatigue and lethargy, and can cause hot flushes and night sweats. During the menopause transition, Vitamin B12 absorption can be disrupted by digestive issues, inadequate nutrient intake and medications that might interfere with absorption.

"The main thing that I have come up against during my perimenopause is fatigue! It's been a bit of a shock. I've always had so much energy and suddenly I'm literally struggling to be awake. Finding ways to deal with this symptom has definitely been a challenge and I'm not ashamed to say that napping has been my favourite option. I'm fortunate to be a freelance writer, actor and director so although I'm always crazy busy, I can organise my own schedule and when the fatigue hits I'll be the first one to find the sofa and grab 30 minutes. Or 3 hours. Sometimes it's not the sofa, it's my bed and it's a full 3 hours of brand new gorgeous sleep. I've also started supplements and really looking at my sleep schedule. I try to get to bed at a good time and wake at the same time because this really helps but I don't always manage it. Mostly, I've learned to set boundaries and understand my limitations so that I don't get overwhelmed. I'm not ashamed of needing to slow down. It just means that I understand what's really important and to save my energy for that."

Anna Friend,
UK (Actor and Author)

TIPS FOR SUPPORTING FATIGUE

- Prioritise your sleep to help minimise the fatigue throughout the day.
- Get a blood test so you can know if there are any issues other than the menopause transition.
- Ensure that you have the following B12 sources in your diet - fish, eggs, poultry, dairy, meat. If you are on a plant-based diet or a Vegan/Vegetarian, you may require supplementation. Some cereals, soy, nut and plant based milks have been fortified with Vitamin B12, folate and iron.
- Within 3 days of using HRT, I noticed an instant boost in my energy and this has been consistent since.

HOT FLASHES

There is nothing more coincidental than being awake writing a chapter on this symptom because it's the exact same symptom that has me awake at 2am! What better way to use my time than to write about it?

I clearly remember the time I experienced hot flashes. They are also called "hot flushes" depending on which part of the world you live in. Living in the tropics meant it was essential to sleep with the air conditioner on. I've always been one to feel the cold so living in a hot tropical environment is my jam. I never needed the air-conditioning to be at the lowest setting (16C) and so a nice comfortable cool room and a yummy heavy duvet would always send me off to a blissful nights sleep.

One night, I woke up feeling like I was on fire. And it wasn't a fever. I didn't feel sick, have headaches or body aches. It was a burning sensation on my skin - like sunburn. That is the best way I know to describe it. It lasted around five minutes and then melted away. The weirdest sensation. During those five minutes, I had tossed off my duvet, punched the air-conditioning down to the lowest setting and wondered what I had been dreaming about to set this fire to my skin. This happened a few times over the following months and by the third or fourth time, I knew it was a symptom of perimenopause. I had begun to research what the heck was going on. Hot flashes was the first symptom that had me questioning what was happening to my body. Sometimes the flashes would pass quickly and I would fall back to sleep and other times, I would be awake for longer and couldn't sleep.

Having hot flashes in the privacy of your bed is one thing, but having them in public in front of other people is taking things to a whole new level. This is where it gets serious because you can be just fine in a meeting, presenting in front of a group, having a nice cup of coffee with a friend one minute, and the next minute, you're on fire, bright red and losing your train of thought. You wonder "Can they see this? Am I red?

Will they notice? How long will this last? This is so embarrassing!". This is the symptom that can send women panicking and off the edge, confused about what is happening to them.

My recommendation in managing this symptom would be to strip off a layer, name and claim it, don't shame it. Something like "don't mind me, I'm the hottest girl in the room right now" or "hot flash INCOMING!" or "give me a few minutes to enjoy this hot flash and I'll get right back to you" or "I'm so hot right now - menopause!". Feel free to use any of these and let me know how it goes for you. My guess is you'll get a lot of blank or confused stares from anyone under the age of 45 and some sympathetic smiles or laughs from the over 45 women, or not, because they still haven't found out what is going on or are in denial.

3 out of 4 women will experience hot flashes and that probably explains why menopause symptoms are so commonly associated with this symptom. A hot flash is a vasomoter symptom or temperature malfunction that is caused by changing hormones. When oestrogen levels drop, our body's thermostat, the hypothalamus, becomes more sensitive to changes in body temperature. The hypothalamus goes into overdrive when it detects the body is over heated and shunts blood away from the core to the skin. This sets off a domino effect of flushing, sweating and the sensation of burning up despite the fact that your body temperature isn't actually rising.

NIGHT SWEATS

I may have been dreaming that I was teaching a spin class when I woke up with sweat running into my eyes, my blankets heavy and wet. It's that real. This symptom had steam blowing out my ears.

I grew up in Wellington, New Zealand which is notorious for sub-antarctic winds that would blow off the water and straight into your bones. Once I began working and earning, at every opportunity I booked holidays in tropical locations to thaw out. This was one of the reasons I lived in South East Asia for 20 years. I love that heat and the heavy warm tropical air. Many people complain about it, but that feeling of never being cold was worth the occasional sweaty shirt and ruined blow out.

Then the night sweats kicked in and it was just disgusting. Not only are your sheets, duvet and nightwear soaked through, but you can't change the bedding at 3am with hubby fast asleep on the other side of the bed. So, you strip off the wet clothes, take a shower, lay towels on the bed, grab another blanket and hope to fall back to sleep, if it wasn't for the cold chills that followed. The next morning, there is the task of stripping the bed and hanging out the duvet to dry, and rebuilding the bed at night just to have it happen all over again.

Oestrogen and progesterone hormones can fluctuate anytime from your mid-30's. For most women in perimenopause, the wildly fluctuating oestrogen and gradually lowering progesterone confuse the body and mess with thermoregulation. Accumulation of inflammation from exercise, stress and diet can also affect your body temperature.

I was amazed by how much adequate and specific nutrition for menopause, and the implementation of an alkaline diet, played in reducing my flashes and night sweats. There are a number of studies in support of a plant-based Asian-style diet (which includes soya and tofu) and research supporting a modified Mediterranean diet for managing the same symptoms. The jury is still out on the effectiveness but both eating styles are anti-inflammatory and predoninently plant-based.

"I'm Australian, 46 years old and I've lived in Asia for more than half of my life. I started experiencing menopause symptoms when I was 39, and my periods ceased at 43 - very young. Living in Asia, there wasn't any outlet for support through medical practitioners or a community. It's not something that is spoken of.

The night sweats bothered me most, because while I had hot flashes, I could manage those. The sweats came with so many things - sleep disruption and the roll on being that I was too tired to do anything the next day, too tired to get up and exercise or do anything kind and good for myself. I really need sleep. I'm not one of those people who can get by on 5 hours of sleep. I need my 8 hours of solid sleep. I was working as a teacher throughout this time and it was a very difficult time in my life because teaching is emotionally and physically demanding.

I was waking up anytime between 2am and 5am and many, many times. Sometimes I would have up to 10 sweats a night! That was not just waking up in a sweat but being awakened by an adrenaline rush beforehand which would wake me and then 10 seconds later, the sweat would kick in. My whole body would be covered in sweat, my pyjamas would be soaked, the sheets being soaked and I would be extremely wakeful after each episode. It was difficult to get back to sleep. This started to impact on my mental state and my ability to manage my emotions, causing me to overthink while I was awake in the middle of the night. I couldn't find anything that would provide relief and I didn't know what was happening to me.

The impact of this meant I found it increasingly difficult to manage the day time activities, and the stress started to pile on. It was hard to find the energy to spend time with my three young boys - 1,3 and 5 years old at the time."

Kim Edwards
- Malaysia (Psychologist)

TIPS FOR SUPPORTING HOT FLASHES AND NIGHT SWEATS

- Implement some of the sleep tips as a priority.
- Eating too much protein close to bed time can also increase body temperature. The process of digesting protein is a heat-generating bodily function. High levels of protein can also cause stress to the kidneys, thyroid, gut and liver. Whilst we want to digest adequate protein to maintain lean muscle tissue, we don't want to ingest it all in our main night time meal. Based on research by Dr Stacey Sims[8], an expert in women specific fitness training, her recommendations for women in the menopause life stage suggest 2 to 2.4 grams of protein per kilogram of body weight. If you are a physically active woman, the higher end recommendation correlates with a heavy training day and the lower end recommendation with lower activity levels and rest days.[9]
- If you are 70 kg, your target protein intake would be 140 grams/day. Aim to get 30-35 grams per main meal and the balance in high protein snacks (nuts, seeds, dairy). This will ensure that you meet the adequate recommended protein values for healthy ageing.
- Introduce soy products, such as tofu, into your diet to replace some meat meals. Soy contains isoflavone compounds that essentially mimic natural oestrogen and no, soy doesn't cause breast cancer.
- Ground flaxseeds contain phytoestrogens so try adding ground flaxseed to your smoothies or yoghurt. Whole flaxseeds don't produce the same effect.

---

[8] ROAR : How to Match Your Food and Fitness to Your Unique Female Physiology for Optimum Performance, Great Health, and a Strong, Lean Body for Life By (author) Stacy Sims , By (author) Selene Yeager

[9] 1 kilogram is equivalent to 2.2 pounds.

- Weaker forms of phytoestrogens are lentils and chickpeas and they are great sources of alternative proteins to meat.
- Have spicy meals earlier in the day if you are a sucker for the spice. Eating spicy foods for dinner can bring on the heat at night.
- Alcohol - for those that like a glass or two. I am hoping you will keep reading the rest of the book after this tip, but cutting back or completely abstaining while you aim to get your sleep under control is the first step. If you are planning to have a drink, then finish your last drink by 7pm.
- Limit your caffeine to the first half of the day.
- Daily HIIT (high intensity interval training) workouts will begin to increase inflammation in your body as your hormones start to change. When oestrogen begins to lower, your blood vessels constrict and become firmer, resulting in a rise in cortisol levels. The thyroid hormones will start to work harder to deal with the excess cortisol. Extra heat is produced any time any function of the body is put under pressure and is needed to stabilise hormones. This is similar to when you have a fever and your body is in fight mode to rid itself of the bacteria or virus. If you need your HIIT fix, break it up into 3x15-20 min sessions/week and alternate with heavy strength training. Heavy strength training and high intensity training is best done in the morning when the cortisol levels are already at their natural peak in the body. If you are sore or tired, don't exercise. Try some gentle movement - a walk, a stretch, some pilates or yoga.
- Let's expand on the "sore or tired" tip - a perimenopausal woman will experience more post-workout soreness as her body struggles to recover from the effort and battles against inflammation and lowered oestrogen. This is your body telling you it needs rest, so rest. Daily high intensity workouts will work against you and your symptoms.
- Integrate stress reducing activities such as walking, yoga, mindful breathing, journaling, and any hobbies that help you to relax.
- Have a blood test for the following: Vitamin D, folate, Vitamin B6 and B12. These are the essential blood markers that are also linked to changes in hormones.
- Vitamin D is a highly recommended supplement. As oestrogen lowers, the oestrogen receptors in the skin aren't as efficient in

Vitamin D absorption as before the menopause transition. This will impact on your calcium absorption which is responsible for bone and heart health. The general recommendation is that women 19 to 50 years should be supplementing 15mcg vitamin D daily and women over 50 should supplement 20 mcg daily. An expert recomendation is that you discuss with your GP the following - your BMI (body mass index), the time of the year, sun exposure and whether there is any history of skin cancer in your family.

- If you have been experiencing gut issues, consider tests for food intolerances and food sensitivities that might be causing inflammation.
- For hot flashes in the work place - speak with your employer about a menopause support plan. This would include sweat-wicking materials for uniform, desk fans and cooler areas to work from as a start.

SORE FEET AND LEG CRAMPS

This symptom is particularly annoying because it directly impacted how much and what type of exercise I was doing. I love cardiovascular training - HIIT, long slow jogs and walks, faster and shorter runs, sprint training on a bike and hiking. I associate lifting my heart rate with lifting my mood and of course it does that! I live for that endorphin high.

I noticed a correlation between teaching a spinning class in the evening and waking up with cramps in my calf muscles and feet. My feet would also burn and tingle, like pins and needles. The cramps would happen when I went to roll over in bed and I would need to wake up and gently stretch and breathe through the cramp until it would melt away. I would manage to fall back to sleep, only for it to happen repeatedly in the course of one night. Once I figured out when and why I would experience this symptom, I removed myself from the class schedule for evening classes and did see some improvement.

As I mentioned earlier, I have always been averse to cold weather. My blood circulation as an ectomorph means that when I am cold, my hands and feet are freezing and it takes time to warm up.[10] It's not uncommon for me to exercise in a merino wool shirt in the winter and never feel warm enough to take it off. If I were to join a yoga class in an air-conditioned studio, my feet would cramp up in certain poses and I'd spend 20% of the class breathing through my foot cramps.

The foot and leg cramps were joined by another symptom - tingling hands and feet. If I didn't wake up in the night with leg cramps, I was waking with pins and needles to my extremities.

There are a couple of reasons why cramps might occur.
- When lactic acid builds up in the muscles and causes inflammation.

---

10 Ectomorphs are typically lean with small bone structures. Mesomorphs are muscular and strong and endomorphs are usually shorter and stockier.

- A magnesium, potassium, calcium and Vitamin D deficiency in your diet
- Dehydration

Decreasing levels of oestrogen cause your blood vessels to become stiffer and lose elasticity and this impacts blood flow. A combination of narrowing and stiffer arteries, muscular inflammation from exercise or standing for long periods of time, as well as vitamin deficiency in your diet can be the cause of muscular night time cramps.

Calcium is also an important element to the muscle contraction process. Without it, your muscles don't contract properly causing muscular numbing and tingling. Calcium is usually associated with assisting bone growth and density but it is also a vital nutrient for our muscles.

TIPS FOR SUPPORTING SORE FEET AND LEG CRAMPS

- If you feel muscular pain, then rest. Allow your body to recover fully. If you know that muscular pain has been the result of back-to-back workouts, then it's time to mindfully recover.
- Consider electrolyte supplementation which supports fluid balance and sweating.
  - Ensure you have adequate magnesium, calcium, Vitamins D and C in your nutrition.
  - Consider HRT. From my personal experience, there was a direct link between these symptoms disappearing and applying my first patch. And yet, I would still advise following the other recommendations.

If your ageing digestive system begins to reject dairy products, you can find adequate sources of calcium in tofu, edamame, spinach, kale, poppy, sesame, chia seeds, sardines and canned salmon, white beans, almonds, figs and rhubarb.

JOINT PAIN

"I think I have a shoulder injury but I'm not sure how I did it" and "I woke up and now I can't straighten my elbow" are just two examples of injuries I sustained while sleeping. I pride myself on housing very few injuries through all the years that I pushed my body past it's limit as a fitness bikini competitor and HIIT Trainer. My two upper body injuries required physiotherapy as the pain and discomfort had an impact on my day-to-day life - working out, teaching classes, typing on my laptop, chopping food and even carrying a sports bag. Both injuries eventually healed, but it was the annoying hip, back and knee joint pain that would wake me repeatedly at night.

I became militant on my exercise regime in order to maximise the training sessions I was doing, without placing more stress on my joints. Not more than two runs per week, not more than one HIIT session a week, yoga 3-4 times per week, and 1-2 strength training sessions. Lots of walking, lots of water, lots of recovery.

The lifestyle changes that I made had a fantastic impact on so many of the symptoms I have already listed, but not so much for joint pain. That pesky oestrogen was causing my sleep regime to deteriorate because of the joint pain I had while lying down. This is where HRT has made a very real and positive difference for me. A few days after applying my first patch, I finally managed to sleep through the night again. It was very noticeable how the pain decreased so rapidly.

> "It all started when I got injured and then BOOM, a myriad of menopause symptoms hit me like a bloody freight train.
>
> Looking back, there were a few signs and symptoms prior to my injury, but holy shit when it came, it came hard and fast. One minute I felt fine and the next minute I felt like I was losing my shit and might need to check in to a dementia ward.
>
> The one symptom that really got to me was the achy muscles and joints. I'm an active, fit person but it didn't seem to matter whether I exercised a lot, not at all, intensely or mellow, I hurt. It got to a point where I was taking ibuprofen daily to cope. Life seemed to have had the fun sucked out of it.
>
> I did lots of research on menopause and HRT and this led me to ask my doctor for help in getting my mojo back. When my oestrogen left the building, my 'get up and go' got up and left too. I felt like an alien had invaded my body.
>
> I now have the oestrogen patches and I have a Mirena IUS for progesterone support. I might add, I got it easily. Within days I began feeling like my old self. My sense of humour and positive outlook on life returned and that was a blessing for everyone. I stopped feeling like I had dementia and I became so much more even keeled - no more suppressing dramatic mood swings! The best part was my body's muscle and joint aches eased considerably. No pain meant I had way more love for life again.
>
> I'm going with thank f#@k for HRT because it works for me."
>
> **Ann Wicken,**
> New Zealand (Fitness Professional)

It's not necessarily the years of high impact exercise that is starting to cause your joint pain, although it can be a factor if your body still has high levels of inflammation, but it's the declining oestrogen level that reduces joint lubrication. We need oestrogen to maintain and protect our cell membranes, encourage cell renewal and maintain and heal our joints. Progeterone levels are also falling and occasionally have surges or "spikes" and these can cause ligament "relaxation" which can often lead to joint injuries.

If sleep is an issue, or becomes an issue again like it did with me, it means that our bodies aren't getting the adequate rest needed to repair and heal.

TIPS FOR SUPPORTING JOINT PAIN

- If you are a HIIT addict and you love these workouts daily, then it's time to change it up. Getting your endorphin fix can be experienced in other modes of movement if you are willing to experiment.
- Prioritise weight training, and I mean heavy weight training, over cardio activity. Heavy weight training is based on your starting point and previous experience but assume 8-12 repetitions per exercise and choose compound exercises over individual muscle groups. If executed with correct form, the benefits to your body from a health and longevity perspective are gold - increase muscle density, boosting and balancing hormones, stronger joints and bones. If you have had no experience or limited experience with resistance training, I would highly recommend some sessions with a personal trainer to ensure you are executing the exercises safely and with the right technique.
- From a nutrition perspective, olive oil is the best choice out of all the options for cooking and dressings. This is because olive oil has Vitamin E, or specifically tocopherol, a natural anti-oxidant. A study conducted and published in the Journal of Nutritional Biochemistry in 2015 discusses the benefits of a compound found in extra virgin olive oil called oleocanthal that has significant impact on reducing chronic inflammation, similar to ibuprofen.[11]
- Include Vitamin E sources in your diet, such as almonds, avocados, sweet potato, pumpkin, sunflower seeds, peanut butter, spinach and hazelnuts.
- True rest and recovery. When you wake up in the morning and you feel smashed and sore, allow yourself to recover. If you need some activity, go for a walk, a swim, practice gentle yoga or stretch.

---

11 http://blog.arthritis.org/living-with-arthritis/olive-oil-anti-inflammatory-arthritis-diet/

TIGHT MUSCLES

As I continued to exercise at a high intensity and teach group classes, I noticed I needed to stretch so much more. If I didn't have a decent stretch or yoga session straight after a workout, I would feel, well, like a 90 year old might feel. I noticed this in my lower back, shoulders, hip flexors and hamstrings. It definitely affected my fluidity of movement. The tightness became so uncomfortable that I would struggle to relax in a chair for longer than 30 minutes. I needed to get up, move and stretch. The upside is that I have made this a part of my life - taking mini breaks between work sessions, moving around a lot more and stretching.

Muscular pain, also known as "myalgia" can affect up to 40% of women transitioning though menopause. While oestrogen does have a part to play in the joint pain one can experience during menopause, muscular pain has a more direct link to inflammation. Oestrogen in the body helps us reduce inflammation and the dropping levels of oestrogen make it harder for the muscles to fully recover.

As we age, bolstered by the decline in oestrogen, our Type-2 muscle fibres which are activated for strength and power, begin to diminish. This causes the loss in muscle tone, muscle size and slows down your recovery from a workout. I noticed that this affected my ability to jump (think plyometric box jumps), run faster and my overall strength. Push ups became harder.

TIPS FOR SUPPORTING TIGHT MUSCLES

- The obvious place to start is to reduce inflammation. Oestrogen is a fantastic anti-inflammatory so having less of it in the body will make your muscles feel tighter and sorer. To support your tight muscles, - maintaining adequate hydration, reducing stress and eliminating inflammatory foods. Yoga or stretching becomes essential to muscular pain alleviation as well as maintaining mobility.
- If you are participating in HIIT workouts and long cardio sessions daily, and don't feel as if you are ever recovering and your body is consistently sore, then it's time for major change to your fitness routine.

IRREGULAR PERIODS

In my late teens, I suffered from debilitating period pain - vomiting and cramps that would leave me on the floor. One of the solutions to manage my cycle and PMS symptoms was to take birth control. This definitely improved my symptoms and I continued with the oral contraceptive until I was ready to have a baby. Once off the contraceptive, I was pregnant within 2 cycles with Jazz. I didn't have the same experience trying to conceive Sol, but that's a whole other story and possibly linked to the fact that I was trying to get pregnant at 39. Let's fast forward to post babies, with Sol born when I was 42.

I don't believe my periods stabilised after having Sol. I put this down to having a geriatric pregnancy. I resumed the contraceptive pill a year after Sol was born and then only used it for two years, until I turned 45. My periods had become heavier and irregular despite being on the pill. They were also longer, anything up to 10 days long - so annoying! And when I had had enough of this situation, I went back to my obgyn who explained the upsides of the Mirena IUS (intrauterine system). The Mirena IUS[12] provides long term, and reversible, birth control. It is a T-shaped plastic frame that sits inside the uterus. The Mirena releases the hormone progestin and can prevent pregnancy for up to five years before requiring replacement. I vaguely remember my obgyn mentioning that as my oestrogen levels start to fall, the Mirena would support me through "this time" until I would no longer be having any periods. She did not use the words perimenopause or menopause - strange, right?

What I did notice once I had the Mirena inserted, was a decrease in periods. The first few years, I would have a period but it was almost negligible - just some spotting and no real symptoms.

---

12 An updated note about the Mirena IUS - if you are 45 years or older, the Mirena can stay in place for 10 years but is only licensed for endometrial protection for 4-5 years.

But then, after a couple of years, every other month, I would wake in the night with extreme abdominal pain that took me back to those teenage years. The pain would last 1-2 days and would be worse than anything I had ever had, enough to put in me bed for the day. I didn't associate this with perimenopause. Again, there was no discussion or explanation of what to expect. I found this chart published by Lara Briden - The Period Revolutionary. The pain and heavy periods - it started to click.

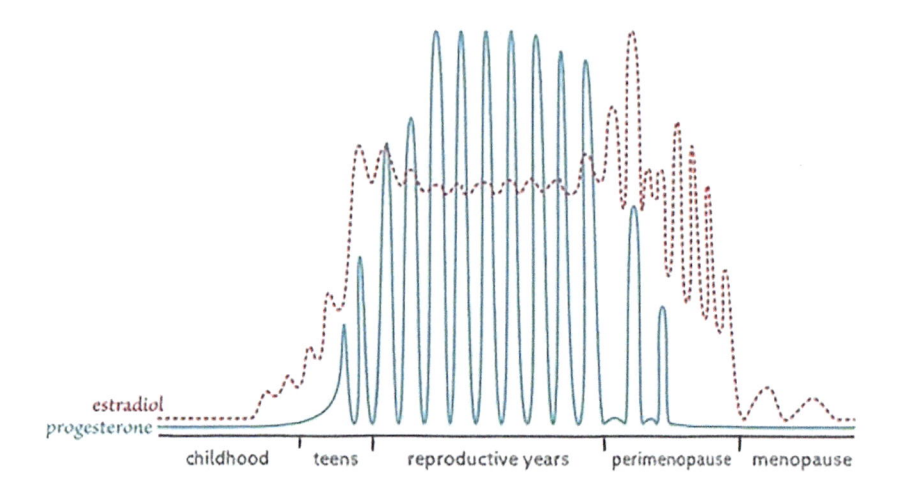

Changes of progesterone and estrogen in perimenopause.

From the diagram, during perimenopause the huge peaks with oestrogen and the decline in progesterone impacts on your regular menstrual cycles. And then it all falls away…

At the time of writing, I am one year away from replacing my IUS. My new GP in New Zealand has explained that it would not be a problem to replace the Mirena and continue with the progesterone support it offers. Great! This makes using HRT easy for me. I have the progesterone support from the Mirena IUS and the oestrogen support from my twice weekly patch. Not every woman can or wants to use a Mirena IUS or any IUS, but I've found it surprisingly convenient with managing my stuttering menstrual cycle as well as the fact that it works in tandem with an oestrogen patch if taking the HRT route.

50% of all women will experience irregular periods. During perimenopause, hormones get out of sync, breaking down the monthly communication between your brain and your ovaries. Bleeding becomes erratic, sometimes shorter and lighter and other times longer and heavier, and can cause menorrhagia (extremely heavy menstrual bleeding). Menorrhagia is not uncommon. The surging oestrogen and stuttering progesterone causes thickening to the endometrium in the uterus which results in those heavy and long periods.

If your periods are becoming scarily unmanageable, speak to your women's health expert on key ways to support this transition. Don't wait until it's too late! There are also non-hormonal medication options for this.

BRAIN FOG

I would get so frustrated when my mum would start a sentence and then not finish and the words would just trail off. I would wonder "Does she think I'm a mind reader?" I would listen in on conversations between her and her friends and they all did it! Half sentences, stumbling over words, lots of laughter. Admittedly, their get togethers were over a glass of wine of two so I just believed it was happy hour that had them forgetting their words.

This is a legitimate symptom. Brain fog kicked in early in my peri-menopause transition and I can see the relationship between the lack of sleep and the inability to string a sentence together. When you are sleep deprived and working long hours, perimenopause is not the first thing you think of as a reason for this.

It was obvious to me during meetings or conversations at work when I knew what I wanted to say but instead, bumbled my way through an explanation of a concept or idea. I started to believe that I was not a good oral communicator. After years of training and educating group fitness instructors, which meant speaking to an audience for 8-9 hours a day, I couldn't string a sentence together.

This symptom is particularly insidious. For years, as women, we work to reach our career goals, juggle a family and home life and then, just when we have reached the peak of our careers, brain fog creeps up and creates a hothouse of doubt. I started to question my 30 year career, and the validity being in a position that I had worked so hard for. Instead of questioning what could be happening to me and if this was a symptom of perimenopause, I tackled my sudden insecurities by emailing my ideas in advance and prepared answers to questions, so I wouldn't feel blindsided.

The impact this symptom had was damage to my self-confidence. I know a lot of women in the workforce will relate to this. I began to have the nagging sensation that I was washed up and over the hill, and that I had nothing worthwhile to contribute. I had lost my words and my voice. I felt that I should just sit down and shut up. And it dawned on me the reason why mature women in the workforce may not openly speak up or contribute is because they may have felt the exact same way. This is an epidemic for women in the workplace. I started to re-invent myself as the "wise one" who sits and listens and thoughtfully answers and only when I could pull a goddam sentence together!

There is relevant research that shows how declining oestrogen affects cognitive performance. The most recent studies by Dr Lisa Mosconi, PhD, Director of the Women's Brain Initiative and a neuroscientist who researches Alzheimers risk to women, show that 80% of women in their menopause transition show changes to their brain. 60% of perimenopausal women are affected by brain fog but the good news is that it's temporary.

" The worst symptom for me during the menopause transition was brain fog. My brain is my biggest asset and always has been. Until I hit perimenopause, I lived a busy lifealways multi-tasking, juggling raising children with work and living my best life. My brain is usually able to grasp complexintellectual concepts easily and also create new original ideas and act on them.

I'm not naturally into physical activity but I know I have to exercise to stay well and I relied on my brain to keep reminding me of this and also organising my life so I have time to work out.

Along came perimenopause and my brain was enveloped in a cloud. I couldn't multi-task at work or at home. I couldn't think aboutanything. It was like living life with the handbrake on. There was no impetus to exercise. I just didn't really give a fuck anymore about anything.

Because I hadn't realised that brain fog was a symptom of menopause, I didn't have a handle of what was happening. When I discovered Dr Louise Newson's website and listened to her podcasts suddenly it all made sense.

I have been taking HRT in the form of oestrogen and progesterone for 18 months now and testosterone for a year. Yesterday I looked back at my journal from the months prior to starting HRT and I don't recognise myself. HRT has made such a huge difference to my life and especially the brain fog. I feel like I am back in vividtechnicolor. I am motivated to move. I have long multi day hikes planned for the summer. I am creative again and writing articles. I am managing work and family with ease."

Anna Sophia,
New Zealand (social activist, counsellor, writer)

In a study conducted by the British Menopause Society[13], 40% of women said they had experienced brain fog and 50% reported to have reduced concentration and poor memory. Changing hormone levels do, in fact, affect brain function. Oestrogen is essential for the normal function of memory, temperature regulation and emotions. As oestro-

---

13 Griffiths A, MacLennan SJ, Hassard J. Menopause and work: an electronic survey of employees' attitudes in the UK. Maturitas. 2013 Oct;76(2).

gen falls, the brain's main fuel source, glucose, decreases by up to 25%. No wonder you feel out of sorts or disconnected.

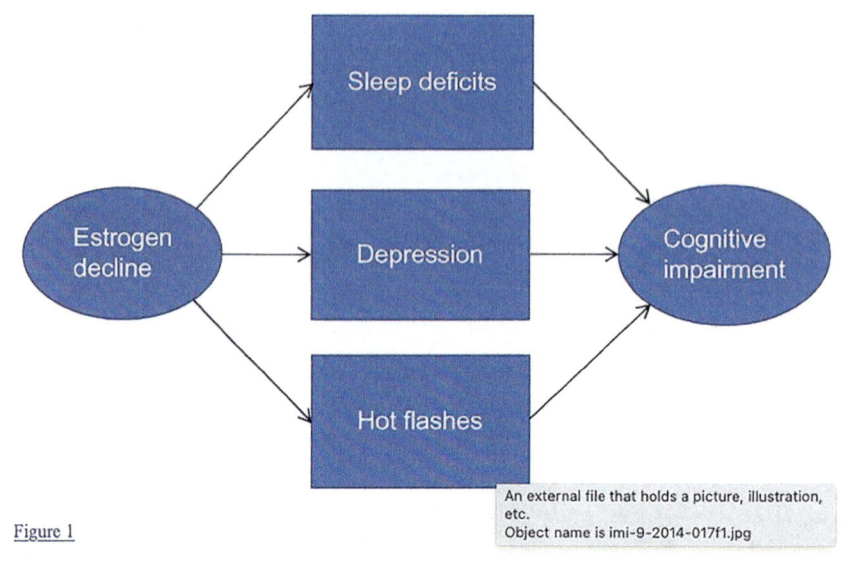

Figure 1

Factors influencing cognitive impairment in peri- and postmenopausal women.

From the diagram, you can see how oestrogen decline affects sleep, wellness, physical symptoms and cognition.[14]

---

14 Memory Decline in Peri- and Post-menopausal Women: The Potential of Mind–Body Medicine to Improve Cognitive Performance
Jim R Sliwinski, Aimee K Johnson, and Gary R Elkins

TIPS FOR SUPPORTING BRAIN FOG

There are scientific studies that show an improvement to cognitive function when you manage your stress, prioritise sleep, exercise regularly, eat a plant-based menu and keep your brain engaged. Here is what I did without knowing that brain fog was a symptom:

- Journal: I started journalling daily first thing in the morning. This was a combination of my thoughts on how I was feeling, a to-do list for the day (so I didn't forget things obviously!), and inspirational words and ideas I was reading. It was my way to remind myself that I was a valuable human contributing to the world and not a shell of my former self.
- Meditation: just 10 mins a day after journaling. To this day, I still find meditation challenging as my mind wanders all over the shop, but I have reaped the benefits of attempting to still my mind and focus. I think of it as brain training and stress relief rolled into one.
- Yoga: I started yoga in my 30's to ease out my sore and tired muscles from being a full time trainer/educator who moved for 9 hours a day. At the end of each day, I would lay down my yoga mat and stretch through the poses. Over time, and with attention to breathing, I noticed that within 10 minutes of my practice, there was a noticeable downshift in my energy and I could almost feel my body relaxing and floating. I felt physically better and my mind was ready to tune out. I've been a registered yoga teacher for a 15 years now and still practice most days.
- Single-tasking: bet you never heard of that! Probably because you've been "multi-tasking" for years? When I realised I wasn't able to multi-task the way I used to and that it was impairing my ability to get anything done, I accepted that a single minded focus would be the way forward. To get a task finished, I will set a 45

minute timer on my phone, play classical music on my earbuds, and keep working until the buzzer sounds.
- Reading and Podcasts: I love to challenge my mind and inspire my imagination. Never stop learning, stay curious, and seek answers to questions.
- Try new things! And then the best challenge I ever set myself was to create a podcast - Sexy Ageing. New hobbies and interests are a great way to take the pressure down while challenging the brain to keep expanding.
- Exercise your mind - crosswords, wordplay games on your phone, learn a rap song! It's the same as muscles on your body. You gotta flex them to keep them strong. Your brain needs that too.
- HRT helped me here! Within 48 hours of applying my first patch, I had my first 45 minute uninterrupted and focused work session in years. I knew what I needed to do and I didn't skip a beat. I felt I had recovered my focus and my confidence started to build again. Note that I had been experiencing brain fog for near on 4 years before I discovered HRT.

MEMORY LOSS

"What was I saying again?"
"What was I supposed to be doing again?"
"Why am I here right now?"

It was so frustrating that I could move from one room to the next with a mental checklist of items to recover and tasks to do, arrive in the room and have completely forgotten what I was there for. And the time frame would be a matter of seconds! We often joke about this symptom but it incredibly frustrating, not to mention scary. When this has happened a number of times and you realise that you need to engage a strategy to reduce it, the "dementia" question raises its ugly head again.

When I think about this symptom and my own mother, I do remember (haha, something I remember), that she started to make notes and lists at about the same age. There would be post it notes and little pieces of paper all over the kitchen, stuck to the fridge, pinned on boards, in a notebook in her handbag.

Up until I started to transition through perimenopause, I never wrote anything down to remember it. But as memory loss crept in, I gave into my obsession with stationary stores and indulged my fetish to find the next best notebook. I had one for the deliverables at work, one for journalling, one for the grocery list and two or three back up notebooks because I couldn't leave the store without purchasing something. I would put my notebook fetish down to a love of writing, and while that is true, the notebooks soon became progressively full of lists and things I needed to remember.

I started to transfer some of these lists to my phone and then, god help me, set alarms for my tasks! I knew things had become pretty bad when I forgot a number of events at my children's school, and started to feel like a bad mother. Forgetfulness was something I was very ashamed of and it caused me great upset. I felt a big part of myself was buoyed in my ability to get a lot of things done and be highly productive. It spilled over into conversations I forgot I had had, and even blurred my memories from my 20's and 30's. Forgetting people's names! My God - the absolute worst!

Here is another moment where I share about my positive experience with HRT. Less than two weeks into the use of my wondrous little non-invasive regulated body identical patch, the forgetfulness has noticeably improved. I have a sense of clarity and focus that I hadn't had in some time and it feels really, really good. I'm not second guessing myself and I feel a level of personal confidence returning. I even managed to win an argument with Dave over who had forgotten to pay a bill, when it used to be me forgetting all the time. My answer this time was "Oh no, you can't use that excuse anymore - I'm on HRT motherfucker!"

Symptoms that I have experienced

"The symptom I really struggled with, apart from the obvious hot flashes and weight gain, was confidence. Over the years my confidence levels had bottomed out. I always used to worry about what people thought of me. I thought I wasn't very good at my job and I really doubted myself. I felt really low about myself and my abilities.

I had been listening to your podcasts and it wasn't until the episode with Dr Rebecca Lewis, the GP from Newson Health in the UK, who talked about HRT that I realised I might be able to do something to help with my symptoms. My partner and I would listen in the car on the way to work and I said to her "I'm just going to book in with my doctor and talk to her about it". To be fair, she had recommended HRT for some time and my push back was that I was worried about strokes. After listening to all the podcast episodes, I learnt that my concerns with HRT were unfounded.

From the first patch, the change was almost instant for me, it was really weird. I remember thinking "OMG - I'm not having sweats and flashes". I've been on HRT for 9 months now and I honestly feel like the old Jenny from before my hormones exited the building! My confidence levels are great now - I'm confident at work, in what I do, in my abilities and I honestly feel like the Jen I was before menopause!"

Jenny Grant,
New Zealand. (Executive Assistant)

Yes, this symptom is real. Oestrogen, the primary hormone responsible for keeping the brain healthy and happy is also vital to the function of many parts of the brain and the way those parts communicate. From finding the right words to taking care of your memory and your mood. When these hormone levels are fluctuating or low, your ability to retain information as well as how you feel is affected. It's a vicious cycle, as the more you feel your memories slipping away, the more the anxiety heightens. This becomes a big issue for women in the workforce as it affects their work performance and confidence. I know this is how I felt, because I was constantly on edge and suffering with imposter syndrome.

Dr Lisa Mosconi, as I had mentioned in the brain fog chapter, has published some fantastic studies that show a direct link to menopause and women's brain function. Her insights include:

The average age for the onset of Alzheimers is 71 years for those patients who will eventually develop the disease, but the brain shows changes between 40-50 years.

Her studies on premenopausal vs postmenopausal women who are predisposed to Alzheimers (where there is a family history) show a 40% decline in brain function.

TIPS FOR SUPPORTING MEMORY LOSS

- A top tip according to Dr Mosconi's research is stay hydrated! Menopause causes dryness everywhere.
- Include oestrogen rich foods in your diet - soy, flax and sesame seeds, dried apricots, watermelon, wheatgerm, beans, strawberries, fatty fish, trout, oysters and caviar! It doesn't even have to be the top shelf kind.
- Ditch the Keto diet - mixed reports for long term weight loss, terrible for your brain health. The low sources of carbohydrates in this diet mean there isn't enough glucose in the brain essentially starving the brain, which is disastrous for long term brain health.
- Limit the high intensity exercise - the stress hormone, cortisol, will cause memory loss and brain shrinkage over time. It's important that we minimise this hormone as much as possible. If you are 40+, reading this, and doing a HIIT workout every day or twice a day - stop now! The recommended amount of High Intensity Exercise for women over 40 years old is 45 minutes in total per week. Your rest and recovery from training sessions should become a priority, so consider other forms of movement instead of the daily 45 minute grind. Your hormones and your body will thank you.
- Brain exercise instead! Crosswords, puzzles, new hobbies! Always wanted to learn a new skill? Now is the time.
- In having suggested to pull back from high intensity daily workouts, this doesn't mean I don't support or recommend physically challenging goals after 40! Life is to be lived and your bucket list - climb Mount Everest, complete a triathlon, run your first marathon - these are important too. Being mindful to your changing hormones and how you can manage them while getting after your goals is living life to your fullest.

STRESS

The double-edged sword - because at any point in our lives we will experience some level of stress or face a situation that impacts how our body has to deal with stress. As women, we have many daily stressors and these often have to do with other people. Relationship stress can come from partners, children, parents, or even friendships. As nurturers, we take on this stress and internalise it. Work performance stress is another aspect, with many women trying to balance everything on the home front while working and maintaining a high level of performance. And don't get me started on lockdown stress, which is something every single person on the planet can attest to. And for those of you who are parents, there is the additional stress caused by homeschooling and maintaining a positive environment without knowing when this pandemic is ever going to end!

There were some specific high stress situations for me that I can recall.

- Having babies, and going back to work soon after. Oh my heart.
- Work travel - and babies - international travel for work and taking the babies OR leaving them at home.
- Losing a job - I was completely blindsided on that one, and was faced with the sudden possibility of having to to move countries in 30 days!
- Starting a new business and all the unknowns that came with that.
- Financial stress of schooling in a country where your children can't attend the local schools and so you have to pay for private education.
- Seeking a diagnosis for my neurodiverse son, and figuring out how best to help him, while wondering what life will be like for him.
- Experiencing perimenopause and not having anyone to talk to about this.

One significant moment that brought home the affects of stress on my body was during a home breast examination in the shower. I ran my hand under my right armpit and hit up against some bumps that I hadn't noticed before. I completely fell apart. I had had a number of events that I can identify as causing extra stress to my life and I could feel the effects before noticing the lumps.

Dave and I picked up the phone and scheduled an appointment the next day to investigate. I didn't sleep that night thinking "It was my turn - I'm 1 in 7". I knew the stats. I am an avid supporter in breast cancer campaigns and events. I have double digit friends that have had cancer.

At the appointment the doctor spent over 60 minutes completing an ultrasound. She told me she could see the lumps and there were a number of them and she couldn't say for sure if it was anything to be concerned about. My ultrasound results would go to the specialist. Five days later (think high stress, no sleep, oh the irony!), I met with the breast cancer specialist who confirmed that I did not have breast cancer but immediately hit me up with questions pertaining to my lifestyle and stress levels. Her questions were the writing on the wall - I had to address the stress and make the changes. A wake up call for sure! Within 9 months, I had two more follow up appointments before the ultrasounds showed no signs of lumps. On arrival to New Zealand, I had a mammogram within 6 months and was given the all clear.

I know you will able to can relate to many of these scenarios and it is what stress does to your body, particularly during perimenopause, that is terrifying. We all know that stress has been listed as a killer for middle aged men, with the classic heart attack that is commonly attributed to high blood pressure and clogged arteries. Women are not immune to this and as oestrogen drops away, our likelihood of heart problems also increases.

When we don't sleep or are emotionally, mentally and physically stressed, there is an increase in cortisol, our stress hormone. This impacts melatonin (sleep hormone) and insulin (blood sugar hormone). You may have heard that not sleeping is the reason why many people are finding it harder to lose weight; they may even notice weight accumulating on the belly, despite consistent exercise and good nutrition. There are studies to show that this is indeed the case.

Excess cortisol in the body also affects progesterone - that feel good/nice/calm hormone. Without progesterone, your body becomes further inflamed and this makes it difficult to sleep and raises levels of anxiety.

With oestrogen dropping off, your body is more challenged to regulate cortisol so it flows around your system wreaking all kinds of havoc. Basically, if you used to be able to handle high levels of stress before, it's going to be a shit show now!

TIPS FOR SUPPORTING STRESS

- Address the Stress: understanding what your stressors are, whether they are young kids, teens, ageing parents, work, relationships, finance, pandemics, and what you can and cannot change, is an important place to begin. Journalling can help with clarifying the challenges. Seeing it written down and knowing that it as a real or imagined factor provides clear insights. I found that some of my perceived stressors were actually stories I was making up in my head. Oh boy, I could take that story to catastrophic levels!
- Having a trusted confidante: being able to consult and converse with a trusted friend/partner or professional helps to provide perspective and emotional support. Feelings of helplessness and loneliness simply compound your challenges further.
- Meditation: learning how to quiet the mind. This is a real skill and it takes time but it truly works! Science supports this.[15] Giving your head space to move away from the stress, helps to calm the para-sympathetic nervous system and lower those cortisol and adrenaline levels.
- Sleep - I sound like a broken record, but get this sorted. There's a reason why this is the first symptom of this book.

---

15 International Journal of Psychology and Psychological Therapy 2010, 10, 3, pp. 439-451
Psychology of Meditation and Health: Present Status and Future Directions
Dilwar Hussain[1] and Braj Bhushan[2] Thapar University, Patiala, Punjab, India[1] Indian Institute of Technology, Kanpur, India

MOOD SWINGS AND ANXIETY

This is an emotionally painful symptom to share and it has been one of the greatest lessons through my late forties and until today.

I value being calm, measured and balanced in my perspective on life which is to know what you can control vs what you can't control. I am an emotionally driven human when it comes to creativity and I listen to my gut instinct on what feels right, and then I do the research and study to evaluate whether my gut is on point, particularly when it comes to business decisions and key life decisions.

When I think back to 2020, I would guess that every human on the planet experienced some level of anxiety. Knowing how stress and anxiety affects perimenopausal symptoms, I can share that I have had moments of anxiety caused by the unknowns of living through a pandemic. There are a number of situations I could write about, but one distinct memory springs to mind. This was the moment where I knew that there was something very wrong but I still hadn't related it to perimenopause at that time.

I was driving to work. A situation of conflict flared up in my head. You know the kind - where you have had a disagreement with someone or you don't agree with their view but you haven't told them yet; you stayed silent but under that silence a spark flares. That spark became a fireball in my head and feelings of rage soared as I went to battle with unknowing individual. The story blew up and I swear brain cells were exploding with the sheer ferocity of the discussion in my head. To be honest, as I write this, I cannot even recall what the conversation or disagreement might have been about. I know I had let it go a long time ago but the craziness of the imagined situation had left a scar. I managed to drive to work and park my car. Once I had parked, a wave of fear and shame washed over me. I was so scared of my thoughts. I was thinking about crashing the car. I started to think about how my family would feel about me dying and if they would be better off without me. I sat in the car and cried over the feelings I had never experienced before - despair, worry, frustration - was I going mad? Was I depressed? Questioning my state of mind shook me to my core.

I did manage to pull myself together but I was very saddened and confused by this experience. I am an extremely proactive person when it comes to my health, and that includes my mental health. This experience was before the movement of being open to how you are feeling and comfortably reaching out to talk with someone. I knew these feelings were not right for me. After all, I had a healthy and loving family, a comfortable home, meaningful work, wonderful friends, but I felt alone and wrecked.

A few weeks after this incident, I approached a friend to share that I thought I might have "mild" depression - here I was self-diagnosing as I often do. I didn't get the response or support I probably needed but then, no one really knew or felt comfortable with that discussion. And in hindsight, I know a lot of my friends and work colleagues looked to me as a source of guidance and strength - how could it be me who was having feelings of inadequacy and fear?

That word - inadequacy - is a dirty little word. It has been the underlying and root cause of all the wonderful opportunities and adventures I might have taken but didn't. As I sit here writing, making my fingers type these words, I know someone out there is feeling all the feels for the times "imposter syndrome" has rocked their world. I know those tears. I know that fear. The doubt and questioning when you have a wonderful idea, dream or goal but you talk yourself down because you fear you are incapable.

Let me share this with you. You are all you were meant to be and more. Your life experiences, your knowledge gained, your successes and your failures have brought you to this place where you are ready to shine and move on in this amazing life stage. That idea, that course, that passion project - the world needs that now. If I can sit here and write and start to build out my dreams of helping women through midlife, then you can follow your dreams too.

Follow your dreams and have one or two good people in your corner who know what you hope to achieve. These are people you trust, who will keep you on the path when you start to move away from your goal, dream or project. They will also be honest with you but they will never bring up those feelings of inadequacy. That can't happen again. You are needed.

50% of perimenopausal women will experience mood changes, anxiety or depression. Knowing this statistic, I am kicking myself that I didn't reach out to anyone and speak about my experience earlier.

It's those pesky hormones again! Serotonin, the happy hormone, is lowering along with GABA (gamma-aminobutyric acid). GABA is a neurotransmitter which produces a calming effect. As progesterone drops, GABA's receptors don't bind as effectively, dragging out the feelings of stress and anxiety.

There is also a strong correlation between anxiety and women who experience hot flashes, but it's not yet known which one comes first. I would think that you would get anxious when you are having a hot flash and then getting a hot flash would make you freak out equally!

"When I first went into perimenopause in my early 40s, I was a bit like a swan from the outside. You would think I was very much in control, but underneath I was paddling furiously. But I was always on time, working hard. I was planned, helpful, confident, and calm. As my perimenopause progressed, my anxiety rose.

I started to panic in meetings, not knowing when to shut up as if I'd lost all my emotional intelligence, leading to painful encounters with senior managers who told me bluntly to shut up and how my anxiety made others anxious.

The tipping point was when I had a panic attack in the office lobby. I was feeling pretty panicky that my new boss hadn't spoken to me all week. I wondered what I'd done wrong and whether I was going to be dismissed from my role, classic cognitive dissonance that accompanies anxiety. I have no idea what I said when he suddenly came out of the adjacent lift. The words tumbled out, I could barely breathe, and he looked at me and just said, 'did you run up the stairs? Maybe you should take the lift next time?". He then turned on his heels.

I cried, and then somewhere in the depths of my mind, a person's name came to me. I googled her back at my desk, and from that moment on, I began to take steps to manage my anxiety. Mindfulness was my way forward, learning to look at my thoughts, slowing down, and anchoring in the present. While accepting for the first time that I am a high-functioning anxiety sufferer, I don't have to respond that way.

Today as a menopause coach, I understand why anxiety happens, and I've coached and counselled hundreds of women, helping them walk through their menopausal anxiety and find peace. Sadly, they are often dismissed, given antidepressants, and even sent to therapists who tell them they have GAD (generalised anxiety disorder). They may have menopause-induced anxiety, which can come out of nowhere, and of course, when we understand what's going on with this hormonally, is it so surprising that we feel anxious? We're having a drop in progesterone which is a buffer against cortisol, so we feel the impacts of stress more acutely. Plus, oestrogen, a powerful hormone with multiple sites in our brain centre concerned with emotional regulation, fluctuates and declines.

The critical thing to recognise is that you're not alone. You can take steps to help yourself like slowing down, resting, relaxing, taking a course *in mindfulness or meditation, or seeking help from talk therapy with a knowledgeable practitioner. By learning to self-regulate, you can become the mistress of your moods and manage your anxiety."*

Clarissa Kristjansson,
Sweden (Menopause Holistic Health Counsellor)

TIPS FOR SUPPORTING MOOD SWINGS AND ANXIETY

The previous tips for managing stress apply here too.

LACKING MOTIVATION

Yes, even this. I understand that there are times in your life where you feel like doing jack shit. Maybe you are tired, need a holiday, need a new job, new everything. This symptom increased in frequency in my daily life and ruined a lot more days than I would like to admit.

I am a list maker - I love them. This is where my stationary fetish is put to good use. I love writing down lists of all the activities and contacts I want to follow through on. The idea I want to bring to life is birthed on a page and then the list starts. It served me well during the worst of my brain fog. I noticed that I would make the Sunday night list and by Tuesday, just 48 hours later, I couldn't be assed to complete half of it. I started to sigh those big heavy sighs, and loll around the house. This all tied in to brain fog, mild anxiety and fatigue - the perfect storm for throwing out the list.

A British Menopause Society survey reports that over 20% of women transitioning through menopause in the workforce experience feelings of low confidence in their performance, waning motivation in their work roles and that menopause had also affected their home life and social life.

TIPS FOR SUPPORTING LOW MOTIVATION

Other than managing stress and sleep, the menopause transition (and I use that word "transition" in a positive way) is a time to review other areas of your life. This was a defining moment when I questioned whether I wanted to continue to work in the fitness industry where fitness is "youthified" and didn't seem to have a place for midlife women. I began taking a review of my life and how I wanted to live the next 50 years.

Here are some questions I asked myself:
- Is the way I am feeling a lack of motivation or a result of poor sleep and stress? I wrote down all the things that might have been stressful, and continued to track my sleep performance.
- In an average week, how many days was I feeling flat and demotivated. Could I pinpoint any scenario that may have caused that?
- What were the physical symptoms of perimenopause I was experiencing and how did they affect my motivation? What was I doing about those?
- What activities have I planned to ensure that I have some joy in my day and something to look forward to.

HRT Update - I remember feeling really energised and motivated after applying my first HRT patch. My to-do list didn't feel so overwhelming and I managed to get through 90% versus 50% or less of it, which also left me feeling more buoyant and capable. The difference between not feeling motivated when you are normally a highly motivated person and feeling like I had regained my mojo made such a huge difference to how I feel about myself and the direction my life was taking.

BLOATING AND DIGESTIVE ISSUES

It's a gut feeling. As my anxiety levels sky rocketed, my digestive issues followed. From my experience, my lower abdomen was feeling constantly bloated and tight as a drum. This was painful and uncomfortable. I know a lot of women relate to this. With regular menstrual cycles, I would experience this for 2-3 days before my periods, but once my hormone levels started to shift into perimenopause, which no one can give you a time line for, I had a consistently bloated feeling for at least 2 weeks! It would even affect my wardrobe choices.

Being in the fitness industry, I worked hard to keep myself fit and be a role model to others. When I was younger, it mattered a lot that I looked like a fitness role model and I do believe the fitness industry perpetuates a certain fitness 'ideal'. I had taken this to the extreme with regular 6-monthly Ms Fitness competitions in my 20's. This involved strict and consistent training and dieting, all in the pursuit of under 10% body fat, a six-pack, visible striations, all of it. For a large part of my 20's and 30's, I was in this condition for much of the year. But I can say, that even with my strict calorie controlled days and low body fat, I still had regular periods. For elite level female athletes, and in particular those on calorie restrictive diets, not having regular periods is a common side effect.

By the time I was ready to have children, I had definitely relaxed with my thought processes around food and calories as I intrinsically embraced a healthy body and mindset to "house a human".

Back to the bloat. I have always been fairly lean but I could see in photos that my lower stomach poked out, enough to look like I was pre-menstrual no matter how hard I tried to suck it in. I suspected that I might have a dairy allergy and possibly some other food factors were impacting on my digestive discomfort.

After consuming dairy products my whole life, I thought I would give it a break for two weeks, just to see how it felt. I also began to research anti-inflammatory diets. The word diet is a bit negative in my opinion because it represents some level of food deprivation. I will go into the diet aspect a bit deeper in another symptom, but I can vouch that shifting from dairy latte's to soy or oat milk latte's with a few other dietary tweaks did the trick. In two weeks, I could see my toes again without having to look over the bloat. When I tell you I cut out the dairy products, that included yoghurt, cheese and ice cream.

"Bloating" can be described as discomfort from water retention and from air trapped in the abdomen, leaving the stomach feeling swollen and sore. Bloating isn't unusual for women as 95% of us will have experienced this with PMS - pre menstrual syndrome.

During perimenopause and the extremes of changing oestrogen and progesterone, our bloating symptoms can worsen and last longer. Lowering oestrogen causes less bile production, slowing down the digestive process causing harder, drier stools. Enter, constipation.

For those with high stress levels and increased cortisol, symptoms of diarrhoea, gassiness and irritable bowel syndrome are common.

TIPS FOR SUPPORTING BLOATING AND DIGESTIVE ISSUES

- As we age, we do start to notice that certain foods don't feel as good for our digestive system. This is different for everyone. Your first line of defence would be to start tracking your food for 5-7 days and highlight the meals and foods that cause some discomfort. You may notice a pattern from your recordings. Take this along to a nutritionist or dietician so they can provide you with science based feedback on which foods might be agitating the digestive distress.
- Note the way the following foods affect your gut - grains, dairy, sugar, alcohol and certain legumes and vegetables (broccoli, cabbage, onions, cauliflower and capsicum).
- If you are constantly feeling bloated and consistent water intake isn't alleviating the problem, reduce your salt.
- Caffeine can be useful as a natural diuretic but if you are experiencing diarrhoea, then consider reducing or eliminating it.
- Add probiotics, either as a supplement or from foods such as miso, tempeh, kimchi, sauerkraut, and fermented and pickled foods.
- If reflux is an issue, cut out the alcohol and caffeine.
- Give your gut a rest. Allow your digestive system a minimum 12 hours, usually when sleeping, to fully digest the food you have eaten throughout the day. Over time, I have found it easier to eat my first meal at 9am (after exercise), and my last meal before 7pm. That gives my digestive system a full 14 hours of digestion and rest. Some might even call this intermittent fasting; I've been doing this for a decade already because it feels good.

(Please note that I am not prescribing intermittent fasting. I have studied the pros and cons but I don't believe that continued intermittent fasting is a recommended regimen for menopausal women)

INFLAMMATION

Inflammation in the body is caused by many things, not just food. Stress, training, lack of sleep and dehydration, to name a few. I definitely had a combination of these at any given time. I am not a certified nutritionist but I had studied some nutrition papers at university to understand the role that macro and micro nutrients play and how they contribute to your health. And of course, the years of playing with my diet to get ready to walk on stage in a G-string bikini for Ms Fitness competitions taught me a lot, too. Without knowing how changing hormones were playing a part in causing inflammation in my body, I had my own little E.T signal.

Do you remember E.T, the Extra-Terrestrial, that cute alien that ends up on earth and Eliot needs to try to get him home? Do you remember E.T's crocked finger pointing to the sky? I have one of those fingers. It's actually my pinkie so I don't use it to point but it is always inflamed, it's crocked, it's knobbly, it looks a bit shit actually. It makes me feel old and like a witch when I look at it. When I'm drinking coffee with a friend, I am self conscious about it. I've even seen it in photos and film.

As my E.T finger started to ache a little more each day and even while I was sleeping, I decided to visit a orthopaedic hand specialist to investigate the deformation of my finger. We discussed my family history of arthritis (my grandmother and mum) and ageing. He didn't bring up inflammation or changes to hormones but I just knew there was a long list of causes to inflammation and my little finger was a daily reminder.

Here is the list of the causes of my inflammation:
- Stress - when you are one of the team founding a new business, there is an immense amount of stress on a daily basis. Anyone who has gone through the journey of starting their own company or getting their business into a place of profit while a team

of individuals rely on them for remuneration, will experience a significant level of stress in their lives. The constant juggling, long hours, whatever-it takes mentality and lack of sleep definitely kick started the stress to my body and mind. Factor in a teenager and a newly diagnosed neurodiverse child and the stress levels sky-rocketed.

- Sleep Deprivation - as per number one (stress), the inability to sleep through the night or the short number of hours based around working days did not support the adequate amount of rest that would allow my body to recover.
- HIIT workouts - ironic that our business was all about this mode of exercise and so being a part of the team meant that I was also teaching a number of these classes and putting my body into a state of high cortisol. Did I mention the brand was called FIRE? Setting the world on FIRE one HIIT class at a time. In one week, I taught 16 spin classes which were specifically designed to get you towards an anaerobic state. A very effective workout but the recommendation for women my age is 1-2 of these…per week.
- Food - dairy, wheat, alcohol, caffeine, meat, nightshade vegetables. As mentioned in the previous symptom, I studied an anti-inflammatory eating plan and started to implement some changes. After 3 weeks, I noticed a significant change to the bloat and I started to feel generally better and sleep deeper.

My mission to reduce stress became an obsession. The more I studied the effects of stress on the body and watched others around me experience the negative impact of stress on their lives, the more I was convinced that this invisible symptom was a fast track ticket to an early death. We often associate the health impact of stress with older men in positions of power - think CEOs and other C-suite executives. The incidences of high blood pressure, heart attacks, strokes and weight gain that I personally know of in men in their mid-40's - 50's was mind blowing.

I learnt that inflammation would have a negative impact on my life unless I continued to chip away at all the things I could do to reduce it.

TIPS FOR SUPPORTING INFLAMMATION

- Start each day with a big glass of water. This will rehydrate your body after that 12 hour fast. I like to add lemon juice because it makes the taste more palatable. There is no scientific evidence to support that lemon in water increases the alkaline effect in your gut. Anything that will help you look forward to rehydrating after sleep - do that!
- Journal, pray and meditate first thing in the morning. Choose one, choose all. Any combination that helps to realign your values and goals and focus yourself. This practice allows you to dump thoughts that don't serve you. Find inspirational messages that elevate your mood, set your mind and spirit to a place that serves your family, friends and the wider world. And, you get to be creative! I have learnt and accepted that my creativity is a gift not to be squandered, so by embracing it at the start of the day, I feel an instant injection of joy that lasts throughout the day.
- Listen to music and podcasts - while writing, showering, cleaning, walking, cooking, driving. Music is like air to me. It is a big part of who I am as a human being - it fuels my creativity. As an ex-dancer and choreographer, I often find myself choreographing movement in my head while listening to music and this leaves me with an incredible deep gratitude that my brain can operate at that level.
- Meditation - I need this in my life. My brain is constantly on the go and meditating just 10 minutes a day has been a life saver. I still don't find it easy, and there are weeks where I lose the habit of it but I know how powerful it can be. The science has shown that meditation can cause a reduction in heart rate, blood pressure and negative stress hormones.
- Yoga - A daily practice would be incredible but I believe if you can accomplish anything for 20-45 minutes, 3-4 times a week, you will notice the positive changes. That feeling of moving my body at a slower pace and incorporating mindful breathing, would feel

like my muscles were thanking me, and I felt a deep calm by the end of any practice.
- Smile at a stranger - it's one of my beliefs that you can give something of yourself every day without expecting anything back, and this one costs nothing. I feel better when I smile. You just never know how that smile might lift someone out of a negative frame of mind. Or they could just think I'm a weirdo but now that I'm past 50, I don't care!
- Exercise or move in a way that feels good to you. As I explore the types of exercise that are best for perimenopausal and menopausal women, I still believe that elevating your heart rate daily is a good thing. I have always been a runner and I was a successful triathlete in my 20's, so running and cycling are forms of movement I still enjoy. I just don't put any pressure on myself to hit a certain distance or speed, and I don't run or cycle every day. It's not a HIIT workout for me. It's a chance to tap into those endorphins and enjoy the fresh air, the sunrise and nature.
- Text or call a friend - since I moved back to New Zealand a year into the pandemic, I left a huge part of my community behind and I feel it. I know the loss is mutual and so when I think of one of my friends, wherever they are in the world, I will send them a text or voice message and if we are lucky with the time difference, we will have a call. And a few times a week, I get to walk and talk with friends with whom I have reconnected since relocating. My friendships are deeply important to me and I am lucky to have these incredible people in my life. Staying connected with people that bring love and positivity to your life is so important.
- Nutrition - I subscribe to an anti-inflammation/alkaline, pescatarian eating method. Not a plan or restricted diet. Much of this is intuitive and there are days that I don't feel that hungry and so I don't force myself to eat on a schedule. I focus on foods that serve my body and mind well each day. I aim to get 120 - 130 grams of protein into my day but I don't stress out if that doesn't happen. I love vegetables and I can literally feel the goodness seeping into my cells when I eat them. As previously mentioned, I have cut out dairy. I don't eat a lot of wheat-based products. I only have two cups of coffee before 10am. I won't drink alcohol

from Sunday - Thursday. Sugar is the hard one for me. Reducing it in my diet is a work in progress.
- Eat no-sugar and no-grain breakfasts. If you are wanting to get adequate protein in your diet, then breakfast is the best place to start. Daily recommended protein intake for menopausal women is 2.0 - 2.2 grams per 1 kg of body weight. Divide that up over the day but try to eat less protein at night to minimise the chance of night sweats and hot flashes. Your largest protein intake should be in your morning or midday meal. I have this incredible smoothie cocktail that is 30 grams of protein minimum and you can find this at the end of the book.
- The following can aggravate inflammation - gluten, factory farmed eggs, dairy, corn, added sugar and artificial ingredients.
- Because I often get asked about what I eat and I want to be as transparent as possible, here is what a typical day, including a morning training session might look like:

Pre-Training: Water and Lemon (500ml), Oat or Almond Milk latte.

Breakfast (around 8.30am - 9.00am): 2 egg omelette with smoked salmon, sautéed greens and avocado - approx 25 grams protein)

Mid morning (around 11.00am): My kick ass clean protein shake - approx 30 grams of protein

Mid day: Protein Bar, 20 grams

Mid afternoon (around 2.00pm): Leftover vegetables or salad from night before with fish or beans/chickpeas/lentils - approx 15-20 grams

Pre dinner (around 5.00pm): handful of nuts and a piece of fruit - approx 10 grams of protein

Dinner (around 6.30pm): Salad or grilled/sauté vegetables with salmon or chickpeas/beans/lentils/sweet potato/brown rice/quinoa - approx 20 grams of protein

TOTAL: 120 - 130 grams. My weight fluctuates between 59-62kg throughout the year.

All of these things I am doing on a daily and weekly basis have come from a desire to reduce inflammation. But it has become so much more than dealing with that one symptom. It all comes back to my desire for a long, happy, healthy and connected life.

LOSING LIBIDO

This symptom makes me sad because I hear women reluctantly sharing how their libido has dropped so much. I think back on my days as a feisty 20+ year old - just thinking, not telling. At the time of writing, I am approaching my 20 year marriage anniversary to my amazing and supportive husband. We had always had a compatible sex life until the perimenopause symptoms started to cramp my style, and then it became a mind game for me. I remember lying in bed in tears after another discussion with Dave about our dwindling sex life and another commitment to ensure we made the time and frequency.

Dave is 9 years younger than me so it's perfectly natural that he would want more frequency, and his body physiology and gender demand it! When we got married, we weren't to know how the age gap would affect our sex life in this way. I hadn't even heard the words perimenopause or menopause when I stood on that beach in Rarotonga and said "I do". To meet Dave half way, I made a mental commitment to do what I could to ensure that our sex life would continue and not drop off a cliff.

(This is a good part of the book to share with your partner).

I now realise how this symptom has such a huge impact on relationships and I would want both parties in a committed relationship to know that your partner loves you and would want to recreate those magic times in the early days, but her body physiology and hormones are failing her - the mood swings, the rages, the uncomfortable sweats and weight gain, even the feeling of not wanting to be touched. You will be the recipient of the negative image your partner has about herself and the fact that she may not even know what the hell is happening to her body. She won't be able to explain it but it will affect her ability to physically demonstrate her love for you. Hang in there! Encourage her to read, research, talk with her closest friends, find a good doctor, have a massage and facial, help with the kids and household chores. The understanding and empathy you demonstrate will build up those brownie points until she can figure out HOW to live with her symptoms and the days she feels good enough to get it on again.

As I write this, I am also acutely aware of some of the wonderful same-sex couples I am close to and how this symptom might impact on their intimacy when there are two women experiencing perimenopause at the same time. I know that women who are in relationships for the long haul want to be intimate with their partners but the lack of libido is a physical and mental, sometimes emotional block. I wanted to show Dave that I loved him deeply and valued the life we had built together, that he was my #1 person. So I put into place rituals that would ensure that I could be in the best state physically and mentally to reciprocate intimacy.

Testosterone, which peaks in our 20's, steadily declines through our menopause transition. The drop in hormones also causes vaginal dryness which has an impact on comfort, enjoyment, arousal and orgasm. Half of all perimenopausal and menopausal women will experience a drop in libido. Think about your group of friends. Half of them have lost the desire to have sex. That's a lot of us!

"One symptom for me during perimenopause that stands out, is vaginal dryness. In my late 40s I started to have a lot of dryness and even pain during sex with my husband. Luckily in my early 40s I had gone to a talk about perimenopause and menopause, so I had a good idea that this was normal.

I noticed that I was worried about it before being intimate with my husband, would tense up during sex because of the discomfort and sometimes even pain and often I was just waiting for it to be over rather than enjoying it.

I decided to go to my gynaecologist to get things checked out, to first rule out another physical issue and to discuss with her my options. She indeed confirmed that this was the issue and shared that it is extremely normal at my age, because of the change of hormones. That made me feel a little better and she gave me a few suggestions, which have helped A LOT...

The other thing I did was talk to my husband openly about it. I shared the issue with him and how it's really normal during perimenopause and menopause and that it was just one of the things we have to deal with. It felt comforting to discuss it with him, so I didn't feel so alone and of course it's good for him to know so that we could experiment with the options and work through it together. What a relief!

My gynaecologist said it's a really important topic because it can put a lot of strain on the sex life of couples and eventually the relationship. It's often embarrassing to talk about, so women typically just deal with it on their own. I wanted to share my experience so other women would know that they are not alone and also that there are things you can do about it.

Angela,
USA, (Teacher)

TIPS FOR SUPPORTING LOW LIBIDO

- Sleep - I needed this to be like a military operation. Tracking through the week would ensure that I was getting quality and quantity sleep to feel generally well most days.
- Communication - regular catch ups with Dave throughout the week, checking in with one other emotionally and having a bit of a laugh.
- Having more time without chores - this included support with household chores, kids organised, no outstanding tasks. Having too much to do and a disorganised house messes with my head. Dave would often pick up the slack to ensure that by the time we bounded to the bedroom, there nothing left on the to-do list to distract me.
- HRT - yes, this did provide the extra pep I needed to have a bed date night. Coupled with no fatigue and higher motivation, it's a great combination to restore intimacy.

INCONTINENCE

Definitely NOT a sexy topic. My first experience with incontinence was postpartum after having both babies vaginally. Trying to get back to high impact exercise 6-8 weeks after giving birth was a nightmare. That's when I discovered Pilates and signed up for one-on-one reformer sessions. The focus of Pilates and reformer classes back then was to help people with muscular imbalances, strengthen the back, core and pelvic floor. Now, it's a trending workout promoted to lengthen and strengthen the muscles, giving you the body of a dancer and as a compliment to HIIT workouts.

This symptom slowly crept up on me. I drink two big glasses of water with lemon when I wake up in the morning. Then I have a cup of coffee. These are rituals I have had for over a decade and they make me feel at one with the world. If I had to be anywhere, teach a class, drive across town after my ritual, I noticed I would need to pee before getting in the car, and again as soon as I arrived at my location. Duration - around 45 minutes. It became a habit that I stuck with and I never questioned whether declining oestrogen levels was thinning the lining of my urethra. And being well past babies, I didn't make the connection that ageing was also relaxing my pelvic muscles. The last time I had practiced Kegals was post baby No 2. I wasn't thinking that this would be something I would need to continue with!

Back in New Zealand and picking up my passion for running, it occurred to me that I would plan running routes where I knew there would be a public bathroom within 30-45 minutes of moving. At first I thought the colder temperatures were the cause of my need to pee. Then I had a an "A-HA" moment where I was able to piece together the information on ageing, dropping oestrogen levels and the effect on muscular strength, arteries and veins. So, it's back to my Kegels. I also had an amazing conversation with Kim Vopni (known as The Vagina

Coach) and set up a meeting with a physiotherapist to check up on my pelvic floor.

1 in 3 women will experience incontinence. Our fabulous hormone, oestrogen, causes the tissues of our vagina and urethra to lose elasticity. This may lead to a sudden and strong urge to pee and sometimes even cause a little leak! Stress incontinence is when coughing, laughing or lifting causes an unintentional loss of urine. You know the line "I laughed so hard I peed my pants"? That is a real scenario. It's also possible to experience more frequent urinary tract infections.

TIPS FOR SUPPORTING INCONTINENCE

- Get back to the Kegels! At the time I had babies, there weren't any funky Kegel apps but there are now. Have fun with that. Pilates is also a great form of exercise that brings a focus to strengthening your pelvic floor muscles.
- See a physiotherapist to assess your pelvic health. We see our GPs and dentists annually so add this on to that health and self-care list.
- Limit your caffeine intake, carbonated drinks and alcohol, fruit juices and tomato-based foods which are high in acid.
- A vaginal oestrogen cream can help as well as providing moisture - 2 symptoms helped with one little dab!

BREAST PAIN

Here is all the titty-gritty on my boob situation. I have never been that well-endowed. I got it from my momma. But that has never bothered me as I've always been active and so my size has served me well by staying put while I moved around, ran, jumped, stretched, you know the deal. And as a symptom when I was premenstrual, I would definitely notice the achy sensitivity a few days before my period.

But during perimenopause this symptom can last for years! There is always an annoying dull ache that doesn't go away. Not enough to bring it to mind as I went along my day but whenever I had to get changed - and sports bras were the worst - take a shower, or exercise, I was aware of that ache. And I swear my boobs grew! How about that? After always being a small B-cup, I was changing my bras to a C-cup. Upside! I'm not entirely sure this would be an upside for women who are already well endowed.

60-70% of women will experience breast pain at some stage of their lives and this is most commonly linked to their menstrual cycle. 40% of women experience breast pain as a menopause symptom.

There are two types of breast pain. Cyclic breast pain is the one you experience during your regular cycle with fluctuations in oestrogen and progesterone levels - like during PMS. Hormones are flooding your milk glands and this causes sensations of swelling and discomfort. The second kind of breast pain is non-cyclical which is more common in postmenopausal women and this is usually linked to a symptom such as cysts, benign tumours, infection, trauma, and fibrocystic changes to the breast tissue.

TIPS FOR SUPPORTING BREAST PAIN

- Make sure your bra is still fitting properly. As I mentioned, I went up a size and I only knew that after being refitted.
- While I never took any medication or symptoms specifically because of this symptom, here are some physician recommended supplements that may help
- Chasteberry: can help to increase progesterone, promote ovulation and regulate your cycles, therefore decreasing your breast sensitivity.
- Black Cohosh: contains phytoestrogens that mimic oestrogen's in the body. Can also help with hot flashes, sweating, mood swings and vaginal dryness.
- Evening Primrose Oil: an Omega-6 essential fatty acid with anti-inflammatory properties that can help reduce breast pain.
- Chamomile: also has anti-inflammatory properties and very rarely produces side effects that some women may experience from the supplements above.
- Omega-3: Omega-3 is a polyunsaturated acid and the most important dietary fatty acid out of Omegas 3, 6 and 9. It is able to reduce inflammation and helps improve bone density. Unfortunately, omega-3 is usually the most lacking in modern diets. The Australian National Health and Medical Research Council (NHMRC) suggests a daily intake of 430mg DHA + EPA per day, along with a 1000mg fish oil supplement. You can top up with the following in your meals: oily fish such as tuna, salmon, herring, sardines and mackerel, flaxseed oil, walnuts and walnut oil, chia seeds, oysters, spinach, soybeans, eggs, marine micro algae and hempseed oil.

Breast Pain is different for everyone and at different stages of life. Just keep checking those boobs, ladies!

ACNE

It's bad enough to experience skin problems as a teenager and it's even acceptable to have the odd flare up postpartum, as one might expect, but to experience acne in my late 40's was definitely on my list of symptoms that I detested. Many of the other symptoms in peri- menopause can't be seen. Unlike this one - it's written all over your face. I didn't get acne, per se, but I did get these noticeable red patches that ran across the top of my eyebrows and down the bridge of my nose and around my chin - the classic T-Zone. They were often itchy, raw and I used a shitload of concealer to hide them away. I began to notice a link between drinking alcohol and increasingly itchy and bright red skin. This was really noticeable with white wine and white spirits. I was in denial about this for years as I loved social drinking and with everything else that was going on, a glass of vino with a group of girlfriends seemed a good way to stay upbeat. And then it had me thinking that I know a lot of women in their late 40's and 50's who drink. I have casually discussed this with my midlife friends and there is a resounding agreement that a drink helps to "take the edge off". Understandable considering.

I bit the bullet and did a detox - you know the kind - no dairy, no wheat, no caffeine, no alcohol, no sugar, no meat, no joy. Actually I am pretty good when it comes to mindfully reducing something from my diet that may not be serving my health, and lo and behold - within 5 days, my skin problems had cleared up. While I still don't eat a lot of dairy, wheat, sugar and meat, I still get the odd spot and dry scaly patch. Damn that oestrogen.

Apart from acne and spots, dry and itchy skin is a very common complaint from women during perimenopause and menopause. The dropping levels of oestrogen strip the skin of natural hydration, leaving it dry and scaly. Flushed skin is another symptom, often linked to a condition known as rosacea, where the blood vessels in the skin flare up and give the appearance of high colour.

Dropping oestrogen leaves the body exposed to the remaining hormones - progesterone and testosterone - which could be the cause of acne during menopause.

TIPS FOR SUPPORTING SKIN CHALLENGES

- Soap will aggravate dryness so using a gentle, non foaming cleanser or moisturising lotion as a cleanser can soften the cleansing process.
- Moisturise skin straight after washing at least twice a day. The moisturiser will keep the water close to the skin and reduce dryness.
- To address rosacea, redness and flushing skin, cut back on alcohol, caffeine, spicy foods and direct sun on the skin. If the symptoms still persist, and they are annoying, visit a dermatologist.
- Protect your skin every day with SPF and a hat.
- Water - lots of it! I am terrible at this one so I set up a water tracker and an alarm on my health tracker.

DRY, ITCHY SKIN

And just like that, one of the symptoms I thought I wouldn't be writing about, rears its head and shows that this menopausal journey has multiple bends in the road. Similar to acne, I am experiencing dry patches of skin on my forehead and chin but worse is the itchy patches on my chest and arms that I find myself scratching in the night. I wake up in the morning to find red welts on my chest - not a good look! Definitely not sexy.

Our skin is comprised of 65% water and the role of oestrogen is to maintain our body's production of collagen and oils, keeping our skin moist and plump. As oestrogen declines, skin becomes drier, thinner, irritated and itchy.

TIPS FOR SUPPORTING DRY, ITCHY SKIN

- I've just listed this but will say it again - stay hydrated and drink more water. Your skin isn't going to retain water the way it used to but you need to provide a platform for moisture for the next tips.
- Moisturise - to create a barrier between your skin and the environment that can cause dryness. Products with fewer chemicals, fragrances and sulphates are better tolerated. Choose natural products with a focus on anti-inflammation and antioxidant properties, that can be applied straight after a bath or shower to lock in the moisture.
- Ditch any products that irritate your skin - these may be products that have antibacterial properties and cause your skin to become even drier. Check in on your laundry detergent. If swimming in a chlorinated pool is a regular occurrence for you, shower straight after.
- Hot showers and baths can further damage and dry out skin. Turn down the temperature and limit shower time to 10 minutes/day.
- If you are planning a soak in the bath, grind up some oats and add them in. Research studies have confirmed that the avenanthramides in oats can aid with reducing itchiness, redness and inflammation.
- Sunscreen! An SPF 30+ can protect from further sun damage and drying.
- Plumping up the good fats in your diet to support your skin from the inside out - foods with essential fatty acids such as olive oil, flaxseeds, oily fish and nuts. Interesting to note that these recommendations are also included as tips for reducing inflammation.
- If you are living in a country that has cool, cold winters, then a humidifier in your home or work space will ensure a skin friendly environment.

DRY EYES

I have worn contact lenses since my late teens because I'm short-sighted. My weak vision impacted me when I started to race competitively in triathlons and I needed to see the buoys from a distance in the water. I started with the hard contact lenses that I would need to clean nightly - the kind that you couldn't afford to lose as these were not easily replaceable!

Over the years, the science of contact lenses meant that we moved from one pair of glass lenses through to monthly lenses and now daily lenses. Wearing lenses became the norm. I wore them everyday for 20 years before I came up against my first issue.

I was travelling and training instructors throughout Asia in my 30's. The days were long and physically intense. We didn't have fitness trackers back then, but my guess, on a daily basis I would burn over 4,000 kcal a day and complete over 20,000 steps. There was sweat, a lot of sweat which meant that most days I would have been dehydrated. Fitness clubs, hotel rooms and flights all pumped out air conditioning that created a very dry indoor environment. I was training in Bangkok, when one day, I woke up and I couldn't open my eyes. I tried but it was so painful that tears started to stream down my cheeks. I called out to my friend, who I always stayed with while in Thailand. She arranged for me to go to a hospital and took me there herself as I wasn't able to open my eyes to see where I was going.

I was diagnosed with "dry eye" disease and given some medication to ease the pain, and recommendations that I avoid the following:

- Wearing contact lenses for 3 months!
- Screen time.
- Air-conditioned or dry environments - which was very hard to do given I lived in 30C temperatures daily.

- After that experience, it was about 3 months before I could wear contact lenses again, and ever since then I have been conscious not to overuse the lenses in order to avoid potential vision issues.
- Gradually, I have decreased from daily lens wear to 3-4 days per week and my eyes feel better for it. I thought I had a full proof plan for managing my eye health when perimenopause nipped that in the bud. Over the past few years, I have had some eye pain, increased dryness and the inability to wear my lenses for longer than 10-12 hours. I now use specialist eye drops at night before sleeping and again on waking.
- Dry eye disease is common in menopause but not a commonly reported symptom from women. This happens when there isn't enough lubrication and your eyes don't produce enough tears causing inflammation and damage to the surface of the eye.

TIPS FOR SUPPORTING DRY EYES

- Give your eyes a break from the screens.
- Use blue-screen glasses - I bought these at the beginning of the pandemic when I realised that I would be spending a LOT more time in front of screens for work and when I noticed that my sleep was disrupted.
- It's hard not to be in air conditioning or near a fan while you are experiencing a hot flash but wherever possible, move away for a break.
- Frequent use of artificial tears. I found the ones purchased at the optometrists were far more effective than the generic brands at the supermarket.
- Drink up! Water that is. You know the drill - 2-2.5 litres a day. Make this your mission.

HAIR LOSS (AND GAIN)

I have quite a carefree relationship with my hair. Even as a teen I was always trying new styles and colours - short when everyone else was long, or dying it platinum blond with pink highlights. I wasn't afraid to change it up when I felt the need to explore another dynamic of my personality. I have coloured my hair since the age of 13 and I still do today.

One area that a lot of women I know agree upon, is that we aren't sure when or even if to let our hair go naturally grey. We admire those stunning women who have a glorious head of slate grey or platinum white hair with chiseled cheek bones and barely a wrinkle in sight. I'd like to think that could be me, but as soon as the patches of grey start to emerge from my carefully coloured coif, I head straight back to the hairdressers. And the frequency for colouring is increasing - so frustrating! When perimenopause affects your hair follicles (and I'm not just referring to the hair on your head), there is hair loss that happens from your head, and hair growth that happens on your face and bikini line.

Let's start with hair loss. I definitely noticed this happening especially as I have quite a lot of length. I have fine, wavy hair and a lot of it, and I noticed when I washed my hair, more and more was falling. I would find hair on my clothes and all over the house and find myself thinking "When does this end? Will I have one of those tired and tiny ponytails?" I was literally competing with my dog to see who could fill the vacuum fastest. Now I understand why older women revert to cutting their hair shorter because the longer the hair, the thinner it can look.

But here is the Catch-22. For all the hair I was losing on my head, eyebrows and eyelashes, my bikini line was making a beeline for my knees and that, my friends, is completely fucked up. Why?! It's not as if we need the hair down there. Or is there a link in the loss of libido and pubic hair heading south to make one feel even less sexy?

It's estimated that an average 50% of women will experience some type of hair loss starting from perimenopause. As we age, and as our oestrogen and progesterone levels drop, our gut absorbs fewer nutrients from our food. This means there are fewer vitamins and minerals to promote healthy hair and nail growth, causing hair to grow more slowly and become thinner. Our scalps produce less sebum which effects collagen production. Hair follicles shrink and thin, and when coupled with an increase in product use, hair colouring and heat styling, the hair condition becomes drier and leads to an increase in breakages.

TIPS FOR SUPPORTING HAIR LOSS

- Apart from the other recommended tasks of decreasing stress, increasing sleep and improving your gut health for nutrient optimisation, you could also try a collagen supplement.
- Collagen is found in your ligaments, tendons and skin. It is a protein and is naturally produced by our body. Some foods, such as bone-broth, have a lot of collagen. Collagen supplementation works by providing essential amino acids to help build the hair's primary protein - keratin.
- Discuss with your hair stylist the best methods for managing your hair to keep it at it's healthiest. Great news for those of you living on the UK - stylists there have access to menopause training to understand menopausal women's needs and challenges with hair!

BRITTLE NAILS

One of the definite upsides of living in South East Asia was the frequency and affordability of having regular manicures and pedicures. My mani would be likened to going out for lunch with a friend. I would do a little pit stop, get my nails done, carry on throughout my day.

I love gel polishes. Nothing beats having perfectly painted nails for longer than a few days, especially when you travel or take a beach holiday and your manicure lasts the whole duration. I noticed that gel polishes started to destroy my nails. I would have it removed after 3-4 weeks to get a repaint and could see that the new polish would last for less time.

The process of removal and repaint actually became uncomfortable and it felt like my nails were getting thinner each time. I can't say for sure whether gel polish was deteriorating my nails faster or whether perimenopause had made its insidious journey to my nails. Over the past few years, if I opted for gel polish, I would alternate this with regular nail paint to give my nails time to recover. Oddly, my toenails only seemed to get tougher - again, messed up. Fingernails getting thinner, toenails getting thicker.

Keratin is the protein that forms nails, hair and skin and is less prone to damage than other cell types that the body produces. When there isn't enough moisture, nails become brittle and dry. The combination of decreasing oestrogen and dryness contributes to nails peeling and breaking. But we know that it's not the only reason. Here are some possible causes:

- Repetitive washing and drying, overuse of gel polish and false nails can cause breakage and drying out.
- Ageing causes fingernails to become thinner and brittle, toenails to become harder and thicker.

- Certain medical conditions may be the cause - Raynards Syndrome, an under active thyroid, lack of iron or certain nail infections.

TIPS FOR SUPPORTING BRITTLE NAILS

- Adequate water intake - giving the body it's best chance to lubricate from the inside out!
- That blood test to check for everything else might also be a key to why your nails are brittle and dry.
- Moisturise - after washing hands and before bed time.
- Wear gloves - for housework and when it's cold outside.
- Take care of your nails - keep them short and manageable, file regularly and use a nail hardener for protection.
- Use acetone-free nail polish remover .Acetone dries nails further.

BODY ODOUR

This feels like the weirdest symptom ever. I noticed that my right armpit was smelling funkier than usual. I detest B.O and I am that person who has no problem letting someone else know if their personal sweating situation is becoming offensive to others while in a group class. If I'm teaching and the air is putrified by someone's odour to the point that I can't breathe and I feel like I'm going to throw up, something needs to be said. Sounds dramatic, but it's crossing the line to mess with my air.

At a spin class I used to teach, a very enthusiastic man would regularly attend and sit at the front of the room. After the warm up, I knew it wasn't just me who was aware of his body odour. Other class members would give him a wide berth, often arriving early to occupy the bikes by the fans and keep well away from him. Some of the members even mentioned to me how they were hesitant to come to class as 20 minutes into the workout, it was unclear whether the air was fit for breathing! I told the members I would approach him to discuss the situation. Luckily for me, the fitness club was doing FREE deodorant samples that week. It was a sign. The conversation went something like this:

Me: "It's so great that you come to the class every week. You are getting a lot fitter!"

Him: "Thank you! I love this class and it works well with my schedule".

Me: "I notice that you are sweating a lot, which is healthy. But it also creates a strong body odour that is noticeable during the class".

Him: "Really? I wasn't aware!"

Me: " That's OK! I'm just letting you know now so that for next class, you can sort it out. And how cool that we have free deodorant samples this week!" I handed him three. Situation sorted.

I think this gives you an idea of how much body odour bothers me, because I am not embarrassed to address it. But when I started to notice my one pesky armpit, I became incredibly self conscious. At first, I thought it might have been an in-grown hair from years of armpit shaving. Then I thought it was my deodorant, so I changed that 3 times. Nothing helped! And I was living in the tropics so it's not unheard of to shower 2-3 times per day.

I would shower on waking. I would shower after my workout or class. I would shower again before bed. And I still couldn't get rid of the one funky armpit smell. This continued for around 9 months before it occurred to me that it might be related to hormonal changes.

That detox I was describing while I was trying to make a difference to my skin? It also had a positive impact on my body odour. I did notice a small difference but the real success in ridding the problem was a deodorant called Mitchum Deodorant Gel. There were probably some powerful ingredients in there that I wouldn't normally use on my skin, but it did the trick! It's interesting to me a year later, I don't have the same smelly arm pit and I am using an organic, metal free deodorant. Sometimes these hormones have your head spinning!

Hormonal changes and body odour changes go together. If you are experiencing hot flashes and night sweats, then you are sweating more which also produces a stronger odour. Higher levels of stress and anxiety - anxiety sweat - is increased during menopause. Decreasing oestrogen levels can affect some women who have higher testosterone levels by increasing the amount of bacteria in sweat and creating more odour.

- Tips for supporting changes in body odour
- I must have tried at least ten different deodorants and antiperspirants before finding one that actually worked! With no endorsement from this brand, I found that the Mitchum gel managed to get my armpit situation under control. For a lot of people, myself included, I prefer to use a natural brand with less chemicals, particularly aluminium, but I only used this deodorant for a few months before managing to get the odour under control. Then I switched back to my natural brand.
- If you are feeling self conscious about your change in body odour, increase your bathing. That will make you feel better but not always reduce the problem. Taking multiple showers a day helped

me for a while, but I was constantly aware of my funky armpit every few hours.
- Carry wet wipes - pH balanced with aloe and Vitamin E.
- Have adequate zinc in your diet - tofu, chicken, shellfish (oysters, crab, mussels and shrimp) seeds (hemp, flax, pumpkin and sesame) chickpeas, lentils, beans, yoghurt, shiitake mushrooms, almond and cashew nuts.
- And magnesium too! Seeds (flax, pumpkin and chia), tuna, brown rice, legumes (black beans, soybeans, lentils, chickpeas), dark chocolate (28gm serving), avocados, nuts (almonds, cashews, Brazil), tofu, whole grains (wheat, oats, barley, buckwheat, quinoa), fatty fish (salmon, mackerel, halibut), bananas, leafy greens (spinach, kale, collards)
- Reduce red meat, garlic, onion, spicy, sugary foods and alcohol, which all increase the inflammation in your body and therefore increase the sweating. It's interesting to note that for the month of "Dry July", I did notice less body odour so drinking less alcohol certainly does seem to have an impact.
- Stick to wearing natural fabrics which allow your skin to breathe - cotton, silk, wool.
- While working out - wear synthetics such as nylon and polyester which pull the sweat away from your body. This helps your sweat to evaporate faster, keep you cooler and hence, smell less.
- Chill, baby, chill - bring on those stress-reducing habits. If I've said it once....

HEART PALPITATIONS

I was asleep in bed and I woke up with a thump. My heart was pumping in my chest and though I don't recall that I was dreaming at the time, I was sure that the physical feeling of my heart racing was the reason I had woken up. It was a bit scary at first but as I noticed my heart rate returning to normal and I didn't feel ill, I fell back to sleep.

There was another time I was reading in bed, preparing to sleep and my heart started to thump out of my chest. Dave was there with me, so I grabbed his hand and asked him if he could feel my heartbeat. Yeah, he thought I was being amorous but one look at my face made him realise that I was afraid I might be having a stroke or a heart attack. This happened a few other times and I would just remind myself to remain calm and breathe through the experience. Because I never had any other symptoms that would have me racing off to my GP after this experience, I shelved it. As I read and studied the symptoms associated with perimenopause and menopause, I learnt that this is one of them. This is a scary one, for sure!

Heads up on this one, ladies. One of the long term consequences of menopause and the effects of hormone levels lowering is the increased risk of heart and cardiovascular disease. We usually associate midlife heart disease as being a male issue but it is also disturbingly high for women entering the menopause transition.

We place a lot of focus on cancer as the major threat for menopausal women, but a study in the UK[16] indicates that women are twice as likely to die from heart disease as they are from cancer. The reason for this is that oestrogen levels can directly or indirectly alter heart beat timing and the effect of oestrogen on blood vessels can cause palpitations.

Lowering oestrogen can increase cholesterol and associated bad fats that can impact the prevalence of heart disease. Putting on weight

---

16 https://www.bhf.org.uk/informationsupport/heart-matters-magazine/medical/women

around your middle (another oestrogen effect) can increase blood pressure and is known to increase the risk of heart disease. That fact alone should be the driving force behind wanting to prioritise our health and stress management over weight loss. Yes, weight loss will help keep the heart healthy too, but the effects of lack of sleep and stress have a lot to answer for in matters of the heart.

TIPS FOR SUPPORTING HEART PALPITATIONS

- It should be a priority to visit your GP to have a health check and rule out anything more sinister.
- Daily exercise - 30 minutes of something that lifts your heart rate and has you moving around frequently will have a lasting difference to your health. If your work is office-based or requires a lot of time at a desk, you are more sedentary. Moving around every hour - a short walk, a stretch - is better than hours of sitting or doing nothing at all.
- Stop smoking
- Consider reducing caffeine for a while, especially if you notice your heart palpitations becoming more frequent.
- Address the stress!

DIZZINESS

I've always had low blood pressure and it occasionally affects me if I stand up too quickly in a very hot environment or after a high intensity workout. I will feel dizzy and my vision will blur.

There was this one crazy time when I was 7 months pregnant and I was teaching group fitness classes in Kuala Lumpur. By this stage, I was just teaching Les Mills BODYPUMP and BODYBALANCE. I had offered to cover a class for a sick instructor but I would have to teach my own class first and travel to another gym for the cover. The easiest and fastest way to get there would be by train. After my first class, I boarded the train and as usual, there weren't any seats available and no one was interested in giving up their seat for a pregnant lady. As I considered myself a fit and healthy pregnant woman and a bit gung-ho, I held on to the overhead strap to balance myself for the journey. When the train pulled into my stop, I released the strap and bent over to pick up my bag. My vision started to blur. I somehow managed to exit the train and make it to some steps where I sat down. There was a minute or so where I didn't recollect where I was. I got my act together and by this stage, I was dripping wet and cold too. I realised I had fainted and attributed this to having my arm in the air for 20 minutes, as well as being pregnant with low blood pressure - traumatic! Needless to say, when I made it to the gym I didn't teach that second class and instead went home to sleep.

My low blood pressure continued to plague me after pregnancy too. When I was doing my yoga teacher training, the studio I was going to be teaching for was offering hot yoga, which was all the rage then. I only had to do one hot yoga class to know that wasn't going to work out. Each sun salutation felt like a roller coaster. Throughout perimenopause, I would get dizzy spells at the most random times doing normal, everyday activities such as standing in the kitchen preparing food or bending over to tie my shoelaces.

25% of women in menopause will report dizzy spells as a symptom. While dizziness can be brought on by oestrogen levels lowering, there are a multitude of reasons why someone might experience dizziness - headaches and migraines, stress and anxiety, hot flashes, changes in blood sugar levels, fatigue, vertigo, dehydration, medications, sinus and ear infections or low blood pressure.

Symptoms that I have experienced

TIPS FOR SUPPORTING DIZZINESS

- Stay hydrated. If you are vigilant about your fluid intake, you may notice that dizzy spells decrease.
- Keep blood sugar levels stable - regular and healthy meals and adequate nutritional intake will help. Do not restrict calorie intake beyond what your body requires.
- Be mindful of standing up too quickly. If you know that you have low blood pressure, then you will also know the circumstances that will cause a dizzy spell.
- As dizziness can be attributed to so many other things, if you experience the following alongside your dizzy spells, speak to your GP - blurred vision, chest pain, fainting, numbness in arms and legs, feeling ill while dizzy or consistent ear problems.

ELECTRIC SHOCKS

This is the most bizarre thing and I wouldn't have aligned this with a perimenopause symptom but apparently it is and I had it! There weren't many days that I wouldn't be "zapped" every time I went to open my car door. It came to a point where I would quickly slap my car so that I wouldn't be unpleasantly surprised every time I touched the door handle. While this symptom may not be directly linked to menopause, there is some support that changing hormone levels could cause Electric Shock Sensations or ESS.

Another symptom, which I don't remember having (haha, don't remember - see brain fog) is "tingling or crawling skin" which can be linked to ESS. The function of the nerves at the skin's surface is changed by lowering oestrogen. This can be related to blood flow and how the nerves send their messages to the skin or a drop in collagen which leaves the skin dry and sensitive.

TIPS FOR SUPPORTING ELECTRIC SHOCKS

- Apart from maximising the tips given for most of the other symptoms, consider having your vitamin and magnesium levels checked.

ALLERGIES

From a very young age, I have suffered from hay fever allergies. When I was a kid in New Zealand, you either had hay fever or asthma. It was like a rite of passage for the freedom of barefoot playing in a park or paddock. It was very common for kids to come back into the class after playtime with runny noses, streaming eyes and coughs . My allergies were debilitating and I was using antihistamines from the age of 10, from spring through till the end of summer.

When I moved to Asia, I didn't touch allergy medication again until perimenopause kicked in but I don't believe the move was the only reason. Every year, there were fires burning in Borneo and the smoke would travel across the region and settle in Malaysia and other countries of South East Asia. The haze from those fires would turn the sky yellow and, because of the overwhelming smell of smoke, we couldn't walk or exercise outside. Many people would wind up in hospital with respiratory issues and my allergies would flare up again. My eyes became more sensitive and I would cough consistently.

During my last two years in Malaysia, and with one of those years in a lockdown situation, most days I would wake up sneezing and coughing. My eyes were irritated and it felt a lot like hay fever again. Thinking back to all the factors that might have contributed to some of my perimenopause symptoms worsening - lockdown stress, homeschooling, no sleep and indulging in foods and drinks I wouldn't have had with the frequency that occurred during a lockdown. If I ingested any of the following - cheese, ice cream, yoghurt, gin, wine, champagne, sugary drinks - within minutes my allergies would flare up.

Fluctuating oestrogen levels in the body can enhance the inflammatory response to our respiratory system. While inflammation is increasing muscular pain, it's also flaring up our sensitivity to asthma and other allergies. With an increase in inflammation, the body will produce more histamines, triggering our allergies.

TIPS FOR SUPPORTING ALLERGIES

- Prioritise an anti-inflammatory lifestyle. Keep those Omega-3 levels high to help process inflammatory bi-products.
- Reduce or eliminate diary products to see if these are contributing to your allergies.
- Vitamin C is a natural anti-histamine - eating citrus fruits, dark leafy greens, broccoli and berries will help.
- If allergy symptoms are not manageable without medication, speak to your doctor about antihistamines.

CO-ORDINATION

This was a tough pill to swallow. I spent my first 20 years dancing. I value my coordination and love to move to music. It's one of my gifts of expression and creation. Little things like not being able to remember a 30 second TikTok dance, not being able to tie my shoelaces properly because it felt like my hands had forgotten what to do, and how I was coaching myself to execute simple physical movements, became frustratingly difficult. It felt like a combination of brain fog and a loss of agility. It made me realise how important it is to keep dance in my life, for my brain, for my health and for my personal sense of joy.

After learning how the whole body is affected by the change in hormones, the sleep deprivation, increasing stress levels and inflammation, it is no surprise that I struggled to tie my shoe laces or to pull the contents of my handbag together.

I chose to to stop judging myself on this symptom and continue to challenge my body and mind. Dance does for me what mind activity games do to keep our brains active. I am still that midlife woman who hits the dance floor hard and closes the club down. My pre-covid commitment to harnessing this passion for dance was a week in Ibiza with one of my besties celebrating her 50th - as you do when you love to dance. And the between lockdown moments in Kuala Lumpur with my girlfriends when we would take over the dance floor and be yelling at the DJ to play our song.

TIPS FOR SUPPORTING CO-ORDINATION

- If you have been reading this chronologically, you can see there is a pattern to how hormones, and in particular oestrogen, affects the body during the menopause transition.
- If you have an activity that helps you maintain your mojo, don't stop doing it. Adjust your expectations and benchmarks on performance, but maintaining your passion for that activity can help with your stress, mood and sense of self worth. Putting aside judgements of what others might think and living your passion is healthy. When those endorphins kick in life will be as it should be again!
- As dance and moving to music brings me so much joy, I make it a regular part of my lifestyle - going out with girlfriends and hitting the dance floor, challenging myself with new styles of choreography, putting music on while I'm getting changed in the morning and just letting my body absorb the beat - this is a huge part of who I am as a person and fuels my mood and creativity.

SYMPTOMS I HAVEN'T HAD - YET

WEIGHT GAIN

Weight gain is one of the most common symptoms related to the menopause transition. I hear from women that they are being so consistent with their workouts, have been the strictest they've ever been with their nutrition and yet the weight piles on. This conversation was a daily with the women I know. I would notice women increasing the duration and frequency in their exercise - daily multiple HIIT style workouts. They'd explore the latest fad diet. The Keto diet and anything low carbohydrate was, and still is, a popular means of limiting calories and carbohydrates to the body.

- Shifting oestrogen, progesterone and testosterone levels all contribute to body shape changes and challenges.
- We lose muscle mass during this transition, and body fat levels increase, specifically in the belly area.
- The loss in muscle mass results in a lower BMR - Basal Metabolic Rate, the rate at which your body burns energy with daily living.
- Increasing stress levels and lack of sleep raise cortisol levels in the body. Studies show a direct correlation between higher cortisol levels and fat gain. Cortisol is an important adrenal hormone that maintains blood sugar, reduces inflammation and regulates your metabolism.[17]
- Hot flashes and night sweats have a correlation to increasing cortisol levels. If you are experiencing these through the night, then your cortisol levels are elevated when they should be low. If you

---

17 https://www.ncbi.nlm.nih.gov/pmc/articles/PMC4688585/

are having hot flashes throughout the day, then you are experiencing bouts of cortisol spikes.
- Note - cortisol is not the enemy hormone. It plays a very important role in the energy metabolism cycle. Just too much cortisol and at the wrong times is when issues arise.

TIPS FOR MANAGING WEIGHT GAIN

- If you have read this book from the beginning till this point, you are likely forming a clearer picture of how weight gain happens for menopausal women. It is a scientific minefield putting all the pieces together. Oestrogen, progesterone and testosterone start to drop and disrupt your sleep. The lack of sleep which elevates the cortisol levels through the night. Elevated cortisol and glucose intolerance which causes weight gain. The fatigue which makes it harder to stay motivated to exercise or exercising while you are sleep deprived and increasing inflammation. So many things happening!
- So with this knowledge, it makes sense to prioritise sleep and recovery as a way to address the creeping weight gain. It sounds so counter-intuitive! A very recent study which isn't specific to menopause but supports the positive effects of sleep on weight loss supports my suggestion that "improving and maintaining adequate sleep duration could reduce weight and be a viable intervention for obesity prevention and weight loss programs"[18]

---

18 https://jamanetwork.com/journals/jamainternalmedicine/fullarticle/2788694?guestAccessKey=e27b8930-7934-4ae2-8a27-c34062f2a947&utm_source=For_The_Media&utm_medium=referral&utm_campaign=ftm_links&utm_content=tfl&utm_term=020722

"I can now think of menopause symptoms that I didn't know were symptoms and how this was linked to my changing hormone levels. The one that had the biggest impact on me was weight gain. And I'm not even talking about a lot. But it was enough to throw me into a turmoil and question why? Being in the fitness industry, being on stage as a group fitness instructor in front of group fitness classes, being a personal trainer and a role model for women...I felt like a fraud.

I had always been able to maintain my weight below 50kg (I am tiny), but all of a sudden, I couldn't! I had this sensational six-pack and then the six-pack became a muffin top. I couldn't fit my clothes and I felt so uncomfortable physically and felt like a fraud mentally.

I felt my confidence and self assurance disappear as I began to lose control of my body. I'm not talking about a lot of weight, but that's irrelevant because the number doesn't matter, it's how that number makes you feel that matters. I felt unattractive, fat and old. It felt like "Who would listen to me, who would have faith in a fitness professional who didn't have her own shit together and was succumbing to the menopause body?"

Chrissie McDonald,
New Zealand.
(Women's Fitness and Health Professional)

CHILLS

We all know about hot flashes but cold flashes or chills are also a symptom. These often follow a hot flash. If you sweat with your hot flashes and your clothes are wet, no matter how many sweaters or blankets you layer, it feels like the cold is bone deep. The chills can last up to 20 minutes.

Similar to hot flashes, when oestrogen drops, the hypothalamus in the brain is struggling to regulate body temperature. Cold flashes can also be linked to anxiety or a panic attack when the body is flooded with stress hormones.

TIPS FOR SUPPORTING CHILLS

- As cold flashes are caused by the same vasometer challenges as hot flashes, there are similarities in how you can manage this.
- Limit alcohol and caffeine as they cause disruption to your body's ability to regulate temperature and sleep.
- Reduce spicy and surgery foods.
- If you experience a cold flash during the day and can get up and move, do that!
- Keep extra layers of clothes on hand. Ironic right? When we are in the throes of a hot flash, we are stripping off and then cold chills have us reaching for the blankets and sweaters. At night, have an extra blanket close by to wrap yourself in.
- If cold flashes are waking you at night, keep a pair of socks on when going to sleep.
- How are those stress levels? Managing stress and anxiety through relaxation, breathing and meditation is a great way to regulate stress hormones in the body that have an adverse affect on body temperature.

VAGINAL DRYNESS

I haven't had this symptom but I have spoken with other women who have.

" I know vaginal dryness most certainly impaired my quality of life. My twenty something self never imagined that thirty years down the track I'd be sharing the story of my dry vagina and how I got my groove back. Yup, turns out vaginal atrophy is a real thing.

I never realised how significantly vulval and vaginal dryness could impact our self-confidence and ability to take on the world until I had a horrific allergic reaction to a vaginal dryness treatment recommended to me in a whispered, almost patronising tone, by a young pharmacist who obviously didn't take 'that kind' of dryness seriously.

I am a confident woman who has always tackled everything head on. I'm not afraid of speaking out, yet the combination of my inability to tell my GP something didn't feel right in a way he could understand and accepting how the local pharmacist treated me definitely impacted my self-esteem. How did I acquire an Achilles' heel in my forties that had such a negative impact on my overall wellbeing? And why was a solution such difficult, un-chartered territory?

Sometimes the discomfort can be a mild irritating feeling when your skin rubs together. Other times it can feel like sand paper grating. You might only feel occasional discomfort at the start of intercourse or be battling recurring UTIs. On a busy day where you're in multiple meetings and running errands how you feel 'down there' is heightening your overall irritability. Vulvovaginal dryness impacts each of us in different ways.

Shortly before my 40th birthday we moved to the edge of the Daintree Rainforest in Far North Queensland, the top end of Australia. We found our bliss where the rainforest meets the reef. Within a year, I would devel-

op sensitive skin and allergies to everything under the sun. I blamed these sensitivities on the unyielding humidity of the tropics. The more wisened postmenopausal me can see that sensitive skin was the first nudge from my hormones that we were about to go on a roller coaster ride.

Vulvovaginal atrophy (VVA) and intimate dryness are a real thing for millions of us as we navigate perimenopause, menopause and our postmenopausal years. Research at the turn of this century minimised the experience of VVA, which was then referred to as atrophic vaginitis. Statistics from the American Family Physician reported that less than 20% of those impacted felt comfortable seeking treatment. While the research has changed, the one thing that has remained constant is we often don't want to speak about it and many of us still do not seek treatment.

Our perimenopausal health concerns and symptoms are finally becoming visible and being taken seriously in academia. The 2020s will be the decade where peri/postmenopausal people are heard. The latest research from Italy where a full Dephi Panel was conducted states:

"VVA is common, with approximately 50% of all postmenopausal women having related symptoms. VVA has a significant impact on the personal and sexual lives and on many aspects of women's self-esteem and emotional well-being."

A 2020 report by the North American Menopause Society suggests this statistic could creep as high as 84% in postmenopausal women and "significantly impair health, sexual function and quality of life."

For me, dryness became a big deal as perimenopause continued. It hurt to use tampons during those heavy multi-day flooding event periods. Afterwards my vagina felt as dry as a dead dingo's donger. Despite the humidity of the tropics, my vulval skin would stick together. My doctor suggested KY jelly - yes, sexual lube! If you receive this advice 'Run Forrest Run'!

Of course using sexual lubricants for intercourse or self-pleasure assistance is fine, but for vulvovaginal dryness lube is not a solution. Avoid KY and vaginal itch wipes like the plague. Numbing vaginal itch wipes mask the problem. Once the treatment wears off you will inevitably scratch. And we all know that once we give in and scratch, no matter how good it feels at the start, the vicious cycle of severe skin irritation begins.

Dryness occurs because of that plummeting oestrogen hormonal rollercoaster. Our ovaries can't figure out what is happening and our vaginal tissue begins to thin and become drier. Our vaginal wall narrows. While this is happening inside, our vulva has changes too, with both the labia majora and the labia minora (the inner and outer folds) beginning to shrink. All this mounts up and can leave you feeling dry as the desert.

Finding the right treatment for my vulvovaginal dryness made me feel sexy again & back to my natural happy self. That happy self is the self we all want to embrace the most during perimenopause and beyond. Treating dryness was the break I needed to confidently shout "I've got this!" to the rest of my perimenopausal woes.

Even if you think you've evaded the dryness symptom, you might unknowingly be impacted by moderate dryness. Trial using an intimate moisturiser. Make it a part of your routine just like you do with facial moisturiser. Apply a vulvovaginal moisturiser to your inner labia as a part of your routine a few mornings a week. You might be surprised by how much better your feel. A happy hoo hoo means a happier you.

Don't let your list of should have's build up like mine did. My dance with sensitive skin from head to toe should have given me an indication that I was at the start of perimenopause and that as peri progressed vaginal dryness was going to be the symptom that would impact me the greatest. I should have had a GP who understood the transition to peri and provided relevant guidance. I should not have struggled with debilitating dryness and be patronisingly told after over 8 trips to my GP "it is not menopause yet, you are just in perimenopause". JUST perimenopause!?! That's where it all begins. Physicians learn in medical school that menopause is when menstruation has ceased for twelve months, but somehow the lecture on EVERYTHING peri and post ended up in the rubbish bin. This has to change. And it is changing every time a woman is willing to share her story.

Many of us navigate perimenopause in a void and on our own. Looking back, my biggest advice if you don't live remote and you do have the luxury of choice is to shop doctors until you find someone who gets you and takes your symptoms seriously. And if not, DYOR (do your own research). Research. Research. Research. Add British author Jane Lewis's book <u>Me and My Menopausal Vagina</u> to your reading list. I wish her brilliant book had been available when I started my perimenopause journey!

Menopause is different for each of us. If vulvovaginal dryness is one of your symptoms, don't suffer in silence. Relief from vaginal dryness be it through a natural solution, vaginal oestrogen, a combination of both, or surgical options will be an integral component of how you manage your *own menopause journey and the years beyond. For me, I took the natural moisturiser route. It totally gave me my groove back."*

Sandy Davies,
Australia (Entrepreneur - HappyPause)

So ladies, you are not alone! I have spoken with a number of experts on the Sexy Ageing podcast who have educated me on vaginal health through the menopause transition. One woman in particular, Shirley Weir, the champion of Menopause Chicks and MenopauseLand gives a very comprehensive and simple explanation of the effects of perimenopause and menopause on your vagina and vulva, and the explanation of vaginal moisturisers versus vaginal lubricants. The use of vaginal moisturisers for vaginal care should be a lifelong investment and should not alter the pH value of your vagina. The WHO recommends a lubricant with a pH of, or close to, 4.5 and osmolality of less than 1200 mOsm/kg. These levels are the same as the vaginal tissue naturally.[19]

Vaginal lubricants are best used to support sexual intimacy.

---

19 https://www.menopause.land/post/moisturizer-vs-lubricant-what-s-the-difference-is-it-okay-to-use-both-day-12

HEADACHES

I know stress headaches - missing a flight or a meeting, worrying about your kids, making challenging business decisions - I could name the issue and then deal with it. Within a matter of hours, my stress headache would leave. But I know a lot of ladies having more frequent and intense headaches and migraines, often for the first time, during their menopause transition.

Wildly fluctuating hormones and an increase in stress and anxiety related to navigating menopause can be the cause of headaches and migraines. Migraines can last anywhere between 4-72 hours and are often accompanied by a warning "aura", or series of visual dark spots and/or flashing lights. Numbing, tingling and nausea are often a precursor to a migraine.

Prior to your period, it is common to experience headaches as your oestrogen levels drop. With the menopause transition, the erratic changes to oestrogen and progesterone can increase the intensity of headaches.

TIPS FOR SUPPORTING HEADACHES

- * Hydration is key. I have mentioned the importance of making hydration a priority in relation to dry skin, skin issues, joint pain and recovery. It's as important here. This may include decreasing and regulating alcohol and caffeine intake if your headaches are frequently messing with your life.
- Take note of any triggers that may cause the headache, whether they be PMS stress, insomnia, or poor food choices.
- Where possible, take some time out to rest.
- If your headache has progressed to any of the following - slurred speech, paralysis in one arm or side of the face, severe agonising pain, and accompanied by a fever, seek medical treatment immediately.

BURNING MOUTH SYNDROME

Sensations of burning from the tongue, inside of the cheeks, lips, roof of the mouth as well as a loss in taste can also be a symptom. Other known side effects include a consistent metallic taste in the mouth and a drop in saliva production causing a dry mouth. BMS can be a consistent symptom or come and go during the menopause transition.

BMS is quite rare with only 2% of menopausal women reporting this as a menopause symptom. Similar to the previous symptoms, there appears to be a link in the drop in oestrogen and even with changes in the reproductive organs, adrenal glands and brain steroids. These can affect the sensitivity of neurons in nerve endings inside the mouth.

TIPS FOR SUPPORTING BURNING MOUTH SYNDROME

- Pump up the fluids. This can help the dry, dehydrating affect on the surface of the mouth as well as cool the burning sensation.
- Cut back on hot foods and spicy foods.
- Adjust your toothpaste to one that accommodates for sensitive gums and teeth. Or switch to the old fashioned baking soda and water combination. Don't swallow!
- Alpha lipoic acid, found in potatoes, tomatoes and spinach, helps with nerve production. This can be found as a supplement.
- There are medications that can be prescribed to treat nerve pain. It's important to note that a burning mouth and tongue can also be linked to other medical issues such as mouth infections, acid reflux, diabetes, or an under active thyroid so consider ruling these out before lumping it as another perimenopause challenge.

GUM PROBLEMS AND DENTAL ISSUES

Declining oestrogen levels lower the bone mass in the hips, spine and the jawbone which can often lead to teeth loosening up and falling out. Gum disease which can cause tenderness, bleeding and inflammation, can also flare up.

60% of women in the menopause transition have reported this symptom. As oestrogen lowers, the tissue is the mouth thins and inflammation increases. Progesterone has a part to play as a bone stimulation hormone so when this lowers you'll also notice that your mouth becomes dry with less saliva production, no matter how much water you are drinking. The decrease in hormones can contribute to gingivostomatitis (inflammation of the gums), bleeding gums, canker sores, bad breath, swollen lymph nodes, fever and periodontitis, which is similar to osteoarthritis for the jawbone. Diminishing bone in the jaw can cause tooth decay and tooth loss. You might even notice that your teeth start to shift around and create more "gaps" between teeth.

TIPS FOR SUPPORTING GUM PROBLEMS AND DENTAL ISSUES

- Drinking water will help with hydration of the mouth and chewing sugar-free gum can stimulate the salivary glands.
- Gums are irritated by salty, sticky, spicy and sour foods, particularly if you have oral sores. Go gentle with the flavours in food.
- Sugar and starch in foods can cause further irritation of the gums.
- Use toothpaste with fluoride, a soft toothbrush and floss daily.
- Dental visits are, and always have been, essential. Twice a year, check and clean.

"I would have to say, the biggest thing in my peri-menopausal journey - everything was so BIG. The tears, HUGE tears and huge sadness at the end of my childbearing years. That was the number one thing. There were so many things but that was the most profound thing I can remember. And it ALL got better too!"

Sally Bartlett
- USA, Workplace Wellness Educator,
Author of "Dammit ... It IS Menopause!"

EPILOGUE

It would be a natural emotion after reading this book to feel overwhelmed, but it's my hope that I have brought some understanding to the changes that are happening to your body and mind during the menopause transition. It's a minefield and the symptoms will continue to shift and change through your journey. Any of the symptoms you may have had or are about to experience are real. It's not just in your head and you are certainly not alone.

I have learnt so much about myself, my body and how I can navigate the next 50 years of this amazing adventure of life. I have learnt to be kind to myself and have a heightened empathy for other women who are about to experience this moment and for those already struggling with it. I have learnt that every women's experience is quite unique.

We are the first generation of women who take our fitness seriously and love the results, physically and mentally, that movement can bring. We are ready to embrace the future with all we know about our changing hormones and we are armed with the knowledge that a long and healthy life is ahead of us.

We are smart and savvy and not ready to be "put out to pasture". We have skills and are open to learning new ones. We have experiences and can help others overcome their challenges with our non-judgemental and empathetic advice. We are smart enough to make adjustments to allow our physical selves to heal and use our intelligence to create new lives on our own terms.

I will never stop searching for more answers to the many questions I have pertaining to healthy ageing and longevity. It's my deepest desire that a conversation on menopause, hormones and changes to our bodies and state of mind will be normalised for all. This book is my small part to play in normalising the menopause conversation.

HIGH PROTEIN, SUPER AWESOME SMOOTHIE (one serving)

1 cup of Coconut Water
1 frozen banana
1 Tbsp Almond Butter
1 scoop of plant based protein powder (vanilla is best)
1 handful of baby spinach leaves
1 tsp chia seeds
1 tsp hemp seeds
1/2 cup ice

BLEND

ACKNOWLEDGEMENTS

You can't get up every day at 4am and write without having a small army of people behind you, waiting for the finished product. Here is mine:

My husband Dave - for his daily encouragement to write and for listening to me talking non-stop about all the things I was learning about the menopause transition.

The women who were vulnerable enough to share their stories.

Mahvesh Murad - for your expert advice and encouragement. I remember the day I told you I was writing. I was cringing with embarrassment and you told me to keep going and then became my editor - thank you.

Emma Barry - the one who was in my corner from the beginning of Sexy Ageing - the podcast. And then you pushed me to reach further and bring to life the ideas floating in my head.

The two K's in my life - Kym Mountstephens and Kim Harvey - who have also listened to my crazy ass ideas and encouraged me to get after it.

Tia Minnoch - my sister, my muse, the most emotionally intelligent person I know. You inspire me on the daily with your zest for life and your talent.

Ann Wicken, Annie Bell, Michelle Trigger and Michelle Carabine - the girls who caught me when I repatriated back to New Zealand. Reconnecting with you after the years and building our new midlife friendships is such a blessing.

Dr Rebecca Lewis - a podcast guest, who gave me my first education in HRT and changed my life. And Dr Samantha Newman who supported the medical advice and science based suggestions for this book.

To all the women who have shared their experience through perimenopause and made it glaringly obvious to me that I want to keep exploring this next stage of our lives.

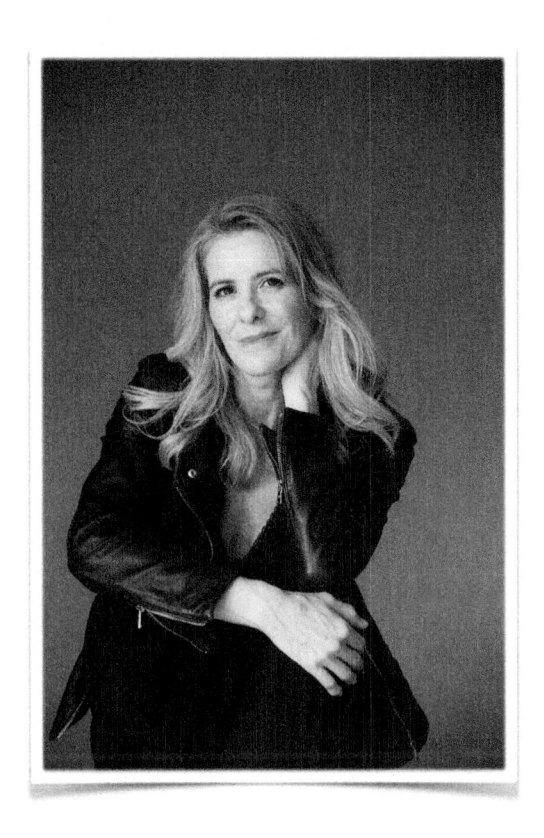

ABOUT THE AUTHOR

Tracy Minnoch-Nuku is a New Zealand based fitness professional with over 30 years in the industry. Tracy lived for 20 years in South East Asia building and working with fitness brands. Tracy has always been deeply curious about maximising life through movement, nutrition and mindfulness, and has applied the science to her own life and to help others. During the COVID-19 pandemic, Tracy launched the Sexy Ageing podcast which became the catalyst to this book. Both the podcast and this book are Tracy's contribution to help women in midlife source credible information and education on the changes that happen physically, mentally and emotionally for all women. The podcast and the book are tools for the reader to ask more questions for themselves and seek support through the menopause transition.

RECOMMENDED RESOURCES

Elektra Health
Cleveland Clinic
Gennev
My Menopause Centre
Sexy Ageing Podcast
National American Menopause Society
Menopause Chicks

Printed in Great Britain
by Amazon